HOW TO TAKE A WA STYLE BATH

FROM THE ONSEN TO THE COMFORTS OF YOUR OWN HOME

WRITTEN AND ILLUSTRATED BY

JODI SAM

HOW TO TAKE A WA STYLE BATH
FROM THE ONSEN TO THE COMFORTS OF YOUR OWN HOME
Written and Illustrated by Jodi Sam
Copyright © 2017 by Jodi Sam

jodisam.com

First Published in 2017

This one is for all the wonderful people around me, and the others, who I have crossed and will cross paths with. My journey up until now has been an amazing one, and am truly grateful of everything.

A special thank you to my parents and loved ones, who have endured me while I was on my own pathfinding, especially Dad. Also to Kanoe for her beautiful calligraphy and lots more. Am forever indebted to you all.

May Love Energy Flow be with us always

CONTENTS

Foreword..vi

Chapter 1
How to Take a Wa Style Bath at the Onsen..8

Chapter 2
Water Temperature & the Body and Other Benefits of Taking a
Longer Lower Temperature Bath..31

Chapter 3
The Modern Japanese Bathroom & the Ideal Bathing Routine..........36

Chapter 4
How to Take a Wa Style Bath at the Comforts of Your
Own Home..41

Notes..li

Afterword..liv

Glossary of Japanese Terms..lv

FOREWORD

Am not a doctor nor a specialist in baths and bathing. I only have a Bachelors of Arts, and that was in International Relations. Why I wrote and illustrated this book is to share with others, who have yet to discover the wonderful benefits of taking a bath, especially *wa* style. *Wa* 和 when used in combination form it means "Japanese" style, method, or way. Yet when used by itself, *wa* 和 can mean peace, friendship and harmony.

I grew up in the modern Western society that often takes fast, quick, and efficient over anything else. Having relocated to Tokyo in 2010 and later experiencing chronic body pain for an extended period of time, I was told to start taking baths every day by my Japanese friends and doctors. I did enjoy the occasional trip to the traditional *onsen* 温泉 (hot spring), but as a person who showered all the time, the option seemed not worth the trouble. However, I eventually gave in during one very cold winter and I have not looked back ever since. I have not been fully cured, but taking baths have helped me with my condition so that I can start off my day refreshed, and look forward to what is in store for me.

Because bathing has a long history in Japan, there are lots of information, customs, trends, what mom had said, and personal preferences, most of them are in Japanese. I have collected what I have known, heard, read, experienced and presented it here in a no-frill format along with my approach to this daily ritual, and hope you too can enjoy the wonders of *wa* style baths!

The following page is collection of beautiful *kanji*, Japanese characters, that were originally handwritten by Kanoe, my dear friend and calligraphy instructor. They are of the main themes that will be covered by this book. Since am not the best of students —my writing and painting skills far outweighs that of my Japanese calligraphy's, she has graciously accepted my request to write the characters for this book that I am now sharing with you here.

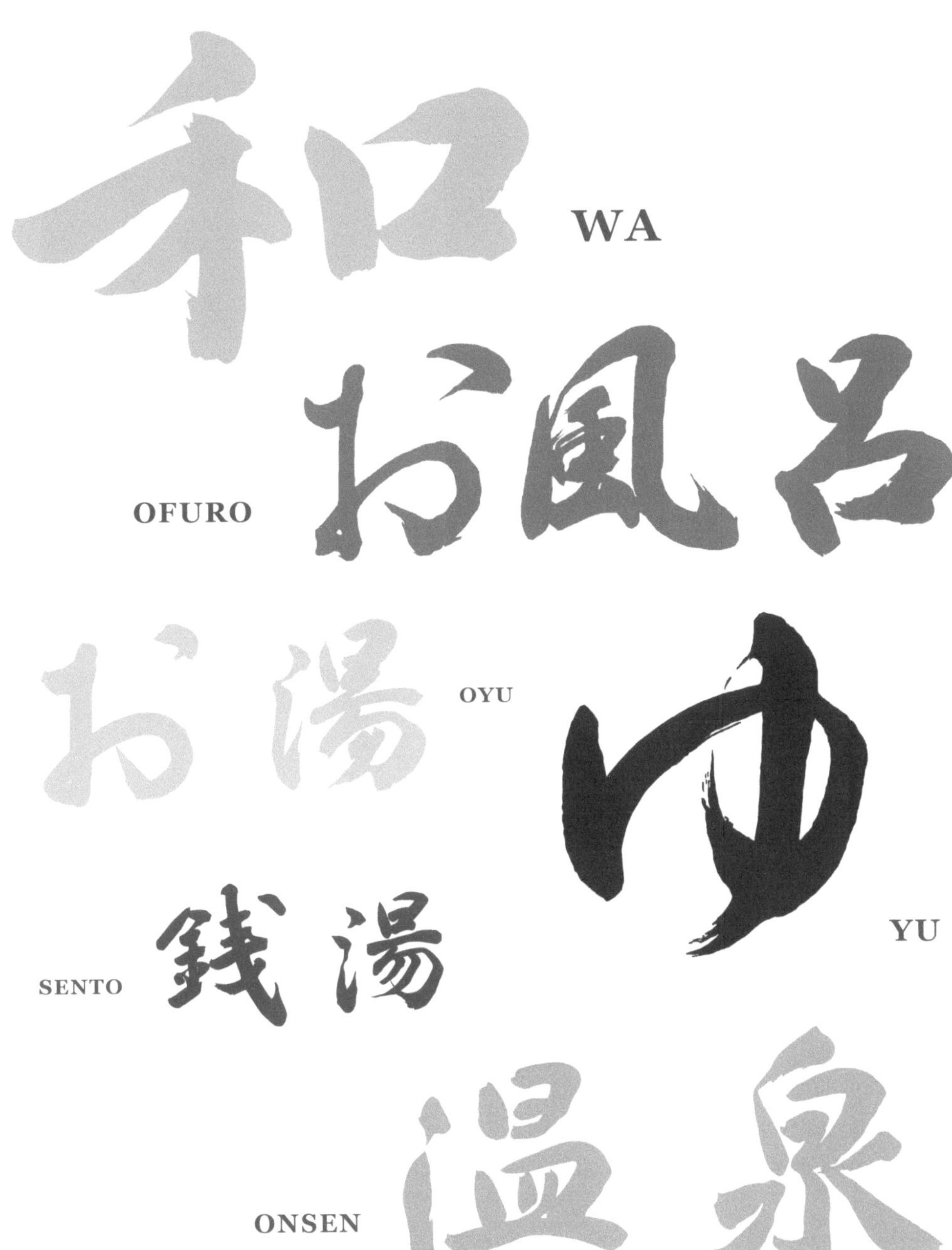

和　WA
お風呂　OFURO
お湯　OYU
湯　YU
銭湯　SENTO
温泉　ONSEN

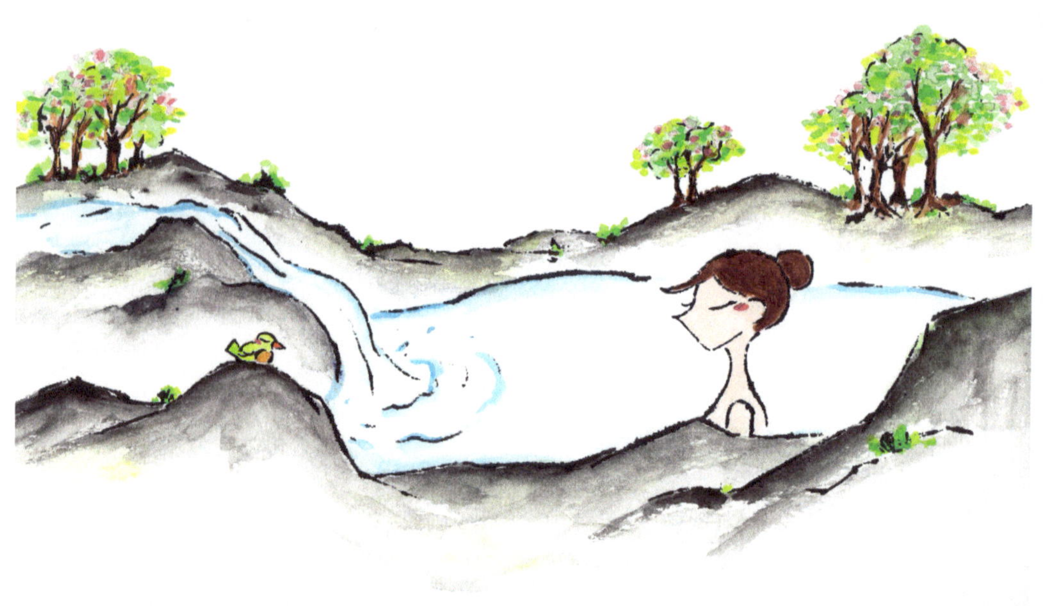

1

HOW TO TAKE A WA STYLE BATH AT THE ONSEN

Throughout history, people have been fascinated by the action or even the idea of soaking in water, be it the Roman Empire's love of big public baths or the idealization of bathing bodies in paintings of the Romanticism and Realism periods, just to name a couple. It is not a coincidence that the human body is made out of 60 - 70% of water.[1] But this book will explore one particular culture's love of bathing, what we can learn from it and, how to adapt it to our busy modern lifestyle, so that we too can reap the benefits of this centuries old tradition.

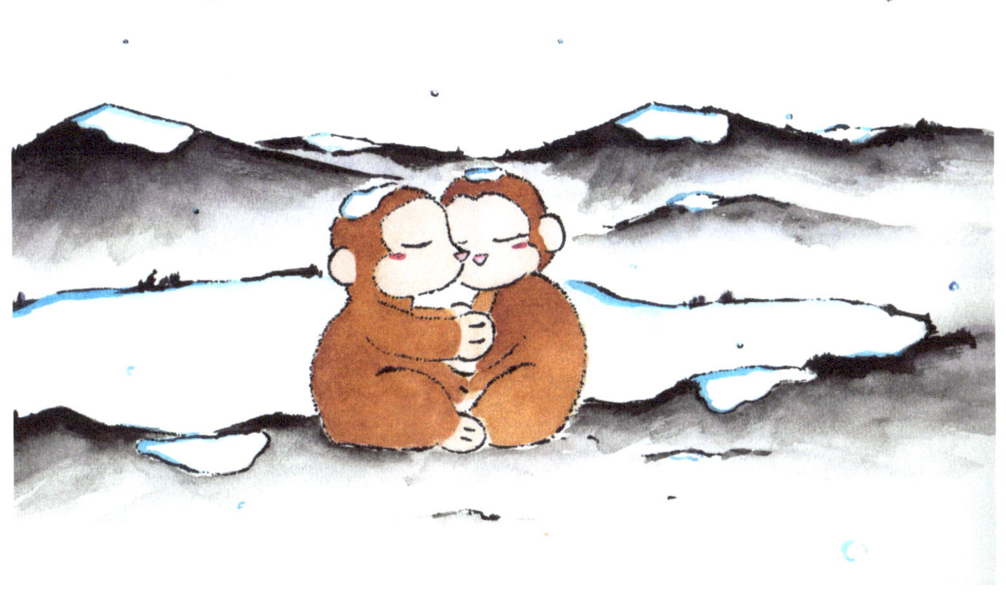

Wa 和 when used in combination form in means "Japanese" style, method, or way. Interestingly enough on its own, *wa* 和 can mean peace, friendship and harmony, which is also a core aspect of Japanese hot springs and bathing culture. Common images of Japanese baths that often come to mind: *yukata* 浴衣 (a traditional bathrobes that are often mistaken for the well-known kimono), *sento* 銭湯 (public bath), Mother Nature's wonderful gift, *onsen* 温泉 (hot spring), and more recently, snow monkeys bathing in onsens too! And how can I not mention the famous ♨ onsen mark that signifies on maps where onsens and sentos are located, or the kanji 湯 *yu* (sometimes with お in front of it, or sometimes written as ゆ), which stands for hot water?

WHAT IS AN *ONSEN* 温泉 (Hot Spring)?

Onsen, is where your fatigue melts and evaporates with the steam, your skin absorbs the rich minerals from the water, and your mind cleanses itself of the day's worries, and the body is surrounded by a supportive, warming force. It is the ultimate reset button. It may sound too good to be true, but for many Japanese, it is a custom, reality, and second nature. If it is impossible to do this every day at an onsen, their obsession with baths at home or the local public bath has got them covered. But let's first take a quick look at what actually qualifies as an onsen and what types there are.

There are outdoor and indoor onsen baths (*rotenburo* 露天風呂 and *uchiburo* 内風呂 respectively), and they are most often found at traditional *ryokan* 旅館 (traditional Japanese inns) and certain resort hotels. These days though, some apartment buildings have onsens as a special facility to attract buyers. Since the majority of onsens are located at ryokans, the reference to onsen in this book will be the ones at ryokans. Onsens also vary in size, from large ones for a group of people to small ones just for one or two persons. The onsens depicted here are of large outdoor ones.

In 1948, the Japanese government created the 温泉法 *onsenho* which literally translates into the "Hot Spring Law". Under this law, in order to be officially considered as an onsen, the water from the natural spring must be over 25°C (77°F) degrees in temperature, and have certain amount of natural chemical/mineral content.[2] This varies greatly from spring to spring. Given the different minerals and in varying combinations and levels, there are over 10 categories of onsens categorized under the Hot Spring Law as listed in Figure 1. These chemical compounds, natural of course, are said to have numerous benefits. It is not rare for people to travel far and wide to soak in onsens with various types of water. Here is a chart of what type of mineral onsen water is thought to be good for which conditions:

Category	Japanese Name	Japanese Name in Kanji	English Name	Known to be Effective for
1	Tanjun onsen	単純温泉	Simple Spring	- Recovery from fatigue, nerve pain, insomnia, hardening of the arteries, high blood pressure, and etc.
2	Nisankatanso sen	二酸化炭素泉	Simple Carbon Dioxide Spring	- Paralysis, muscle/joint pain, contusions, high blood pressure, hardening of the arteries, cuts, sensitivity to cold, menopausal disorders, infertility, and etc.

FIG 1. *(Continued on Page 11)*

Category	Japanese Name	Japanese Name in Kanji	English Name	Known to be Effective for
3	Tansansuiso ensen	炭酸水素塩泉	Bicarbonated Earth Spring (Carbonated)	- Muscle/joint pain, contusions, cuts, chronic skin diseases, and etc.
4	Enkabutsusen	塩化物泉	Sodium Bicarbonated Spring (Carbonated)	- Muscle/joint pain, contusions, cuts, chronic skin diseases, and etc.
5	Gan yososen	含よう素泉	Chloride Spring	- Muscle/joint pain, contusions, sprains, sensitivity to cold, chronic women's diseases, infertility, and etc.
6	Ryusan ensen	硫酸塩泉	Sulphate Spring	- Calcium Sulphate Spring: Rheumatism, bruises, cuts, burns, and etc. - Sodium Sulphate Spring: High blood pressure, hardening of the arteries, external wounds, and etc. - Magnesium Sulphate Spring: Same as the two other Sulphate noted above
7	Gan tetsusen	含鉄泉	Ferruginous Spring	- Anemia, rheumatism, menopausal disorders, hypoplastic uterus, chronic eczema, and etc.
8	Iosen	硫黄泉	Sulphur Spring	- High blood pressure, hardening of the arteries, chronic skin diseases, joint pain, and etc.
9	Sanseisen	酸性泉	Acidic Spring	- Chronic skin diseases, chronic women's diseases, diabetes, athlete's foot, and etc.
10	Hoshanosen	放射能泉	Radioactive Spring	- High blood pressure, hardening of the arteries, nerve pain, rheumatism, calming stress, gout, and etc.

FIG 1. CATEGORIES OF ONSEN AND THEIR PROPERTIES[3]

Note: Carbonated, meaning with natural gas bubbles in the water. And yes, you read correctly, Radioactive Spring, but the minuscule amount of radiation coming from the water is not enough to cause bodily harm to bathers, and the radiation dissipates once you leave the water. For those who are interested in finding more about the the the properties of the various onsen water, I encourage you to visit the The Japan Health & Research Institute's website for more information.

Onsen bathers who are particular about the source of the spring, onsen can be further categorized by the system of how the water is released into the baths, and how water is or not treated. Here is an overview chart of the 5 categories (Figure 2). Only the first two categories have a specific Japanese term name, the rest have descriptive names.

Onsens can be enjoyed privately if you are lucky to have one in your ryokan room, or if your ryokan have onsens for bathers to "borrow" for a limited amount of time, *kashikiri onsen* 貸切温泉. However, in most cases, onsen is enjoyed with others, so let's now turn to the customs or the "proper way" of enjoying a traditional onsen.

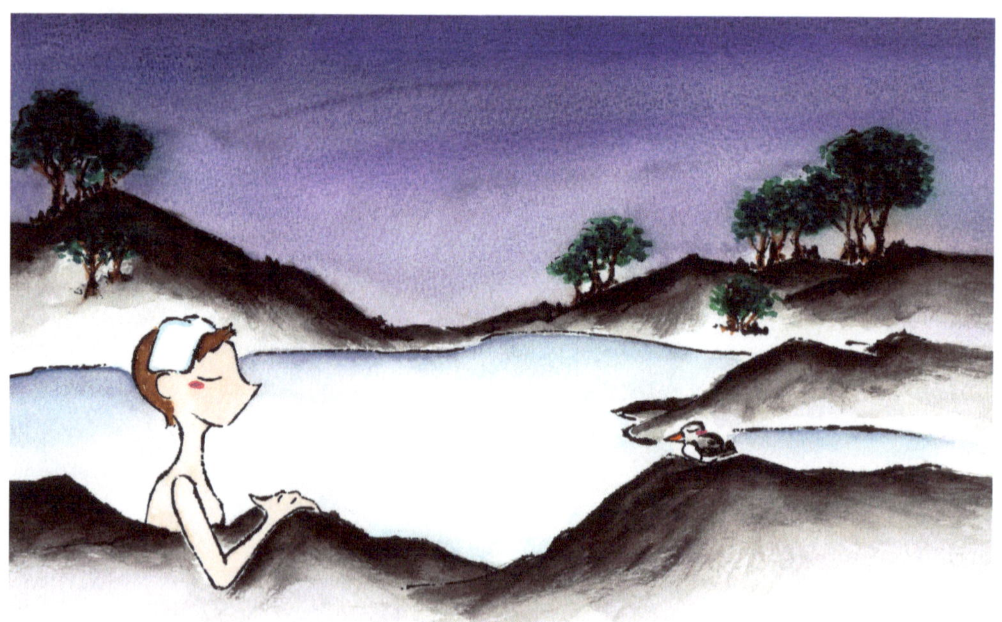

ENJOYING AN OUTDOOR ONSEN AT NIGHT

Japanese Name	Japanese Name in Kanji	English Name	Characteristics
Gensen kakenagashi	源泉かけ流し	Continuous flow from source	- No water added to source water (hot spring supply) - Heat may be added if source water is low in temperature - With high temperature source water, the temperature is adjusted by the use of heat-exchange devices either at the point where the water enters the bath, or in the bath itself. - Water is always released without using a circulation system
Kakenagashi	かけ流し	Continuous flow	- Both water and heat are added to the source water to make it more suitable for bathing - Water does not go through a circulation system
Kyutoguchi gensen - Yokuso kaon junkan	給湯口源泉・浴槽加温循環	Direct flow from source - heated and circulation bath system	- The source water is untouched at the entry point - A circulation system is used to maintain a suitable water temperature
Kyutoguchi gensen - Yokuso kaon - Roka - Sakkin junkan	給湯口源泉・浴槽加温・濾過・殺菌循環	Direct flow from source - heated, filtered, sterilized, and circulation system	- The hot spring supply is untreated as it enters the bath from the entry point - A circulation system is used to heat the water to maintain a suitable temperature - Water is purified and sterilized while being circulated
Kyutoguchi wo fukumu kaon - Roka - Sakkin junkan	給湯口を含む加温・濾過・殺菌循環	Hot spring supply is heated, filtered and sterilized before entering the bath	- Prior to releasing into the bath, the water is ran through a circulation system that is used to maintain a suitable temperature - Water is purified and sterilized beforehand

Fig. 2 further categories of onsen water[4]

ENJOYING ONSENS

"Dai Yokujo" The Bathing Area
How do you enjoy onsens, you ask? Well, onsen water is usually channelled into a ryokan or hotel's *dai yokujo* 大浴場 or bathing area, which consists of: a changing room, washing area, and big baths (open-air bath, indoor bath, or both).

The bathing area is usually separated into two sections and by gender—ladies and men. This is clearly marked by a *noren* のれん, Japanese short split curtains or curtain dividers, with *onna* 女 (woman) and *otoko* 男 (man) kanji characters written on them. And in many places, the gender usage of onsen changes according to the time of the day. For example, a ryokan that has 2 bathing sections with 2 to 3 different types of baths each. Ladies would use Bathing Area A from late afternoon to midnight, while men would use Bathing Area B during the same time. On the early morning of the next

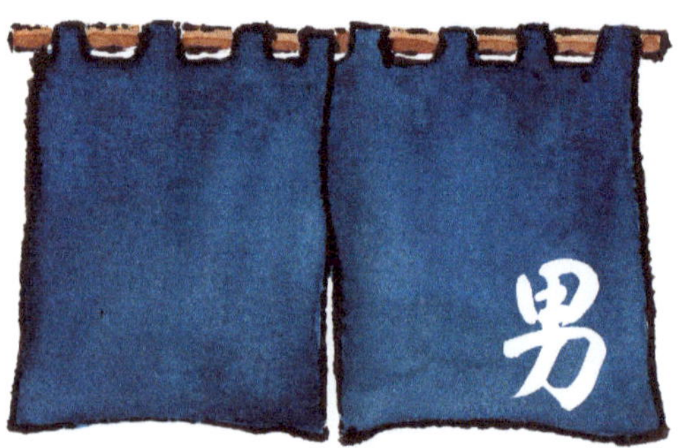

NOREN FOR MEN

NOREN FOR LADIES

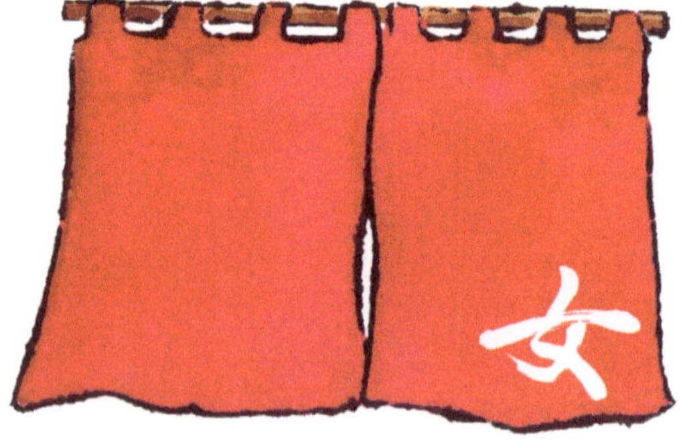

day, ladies would use Bathing Area B and men would use Area A until noon. This way, both ladies and men would be able to try all the different and wonderful baths the ryokan has to offer. There are some places where unisex baths, *konyoku* 混浴 (note, the changing rooms and showering areas remain separated) still exist and are enjoyed by both ladies and men at the same time.

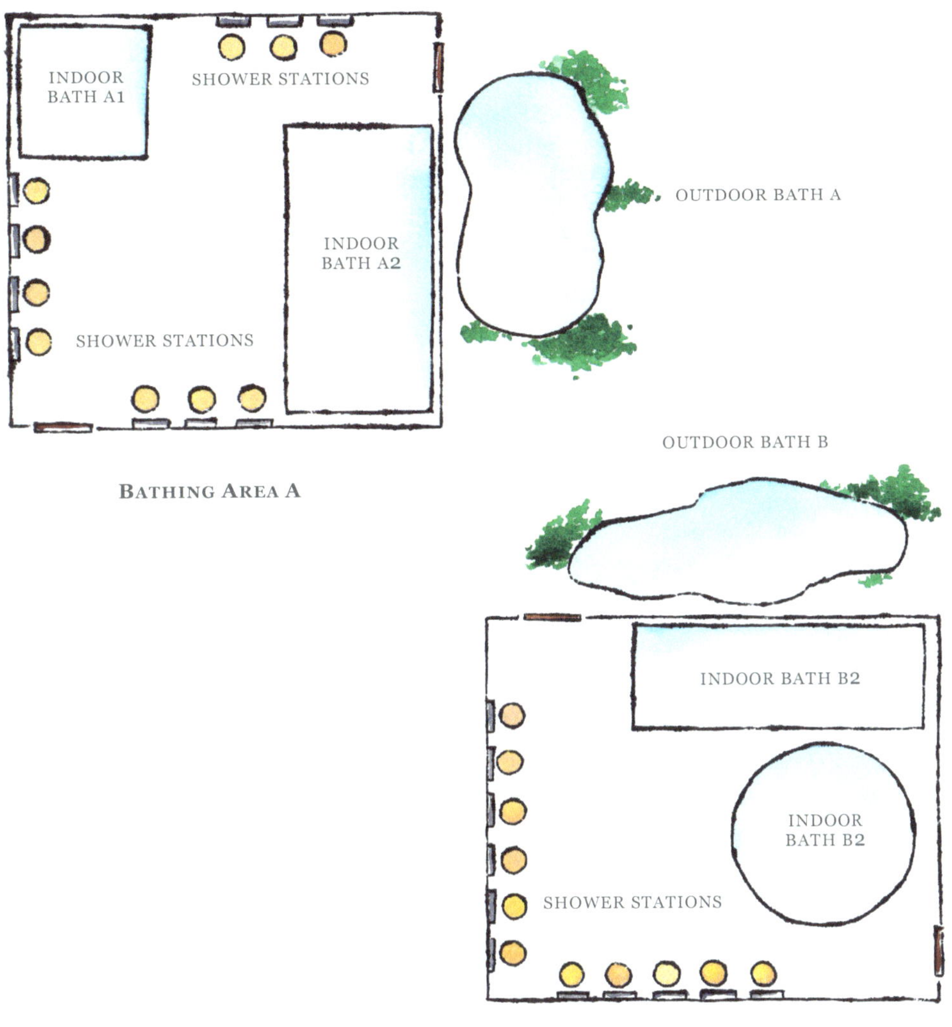

BATHING AREA A

BATHING AREA B

Street shoes or even indoor slippers are not permitted into the bathing area, including the changing room. It is customary to remove your shoes or slippers near the entrance, where there is a shoe cabinet provided. Now you have entered the bathing area, you will be in the changing room, *datsui jo* 脱衣所.

But before we move on, hydration is essential, so please remember to have some water before entering the changing room. It is said that a person usually loses approximately 500 mL of fluid from taking just regular bath, and without proper hydration, the blood thickens, causing what can be a dangerous slowdown in blood circulation.[5] In order to prevent this from happening, rehydrate plentifully around 15 minutes beforehand, since that is the amount it takes for the fluid to travel throughout the body.[6] I personally recommend bringing a bottle of water with you that you can leave in cabinets, or at times baskets, in changing area just in case if there is no drinking water available nearby. Though eating and drinking is prohibited in the washing area and baths, you never know when you need to rehydrate yourself quickly, especially if it is your first time visiting an onsen.

Changing
About changing, it is a custom to bathe without any garments (swimsuits, robes, and etc.). Yes, it can be embarrassing at first, but once you entered the onsen, it is so relaxing and calm that most of your initial worries and embarrassment will disappear. Only in some rare cases, for example at some small number of unisex baths or for the filming of TV productions, where special robes and towels are ever allowed.

There are usually plenty of towels provided to the bathers, sometimes at a charge, so you will not be walking around stark naked per se. But do remember that the towels are not meant to be used as a coverup robe while soaking in the onsen, as they should not be fully immersed in water. This is also why there are many images depicting bathers with towels on top of their heads. They keep their towels with them, without the towels getting wet, and they can use the towels to cover themselves as soon as they get up to leave a bath. However, many bathers just carry their towels with them and leave the towels close by.

Washing
Why must you wash before entering a bath? For sanitary reasons and for the respect of other users who are also using the water, this is an old tradition that has been

followed by bathers. Yes, onsen water is not washing or cleansing water but soaking water to be shared with others, and unlike swimming pool water, it is normally not sterilized with harsh chemicals. The purer the water, the more prized it is. This actually carries over to modern day Japanese bathing habits at home, where each member of the family will take turns, showering and then soaking in the bath, with the same bath water being used by the entire family.

You are required: to remove your make-up (if you have any on), take off all your clothes (yes, all as mentioned above) and jewellery, since some of the minerals in the water may react with or discolour them, and wash yourself at the open communal washing/showering space (*arai ba* 洗い場), which to the surprise of most from other cultures, is really wide open without any walls or dividers. Shampoo, conditioner, and soap are provided, so there will be no need to bring your own. They are individual "shower stations" so to say.

I say showering, but it is usually just the shower head with a short hose attached to a water faucet, and it is really low, approximately knee-high in height. It is made so that

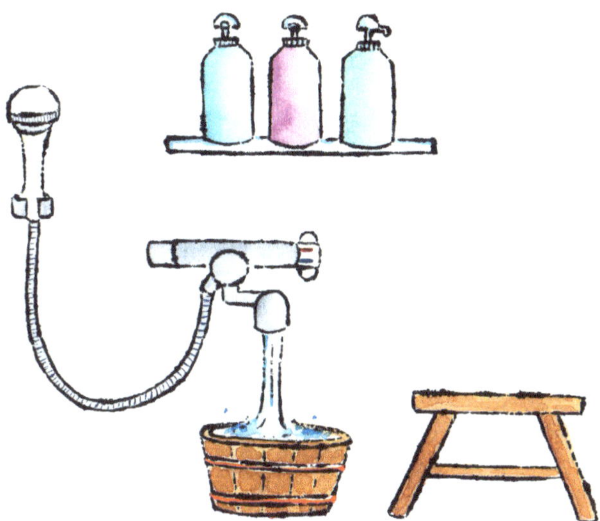

A TYPICAL SHOWER STATION: SHAMPOO, CONDITIONER, BODY SOAP, A LOWER SHOWER HEAD, FAUCET, BUCKET & STOOL

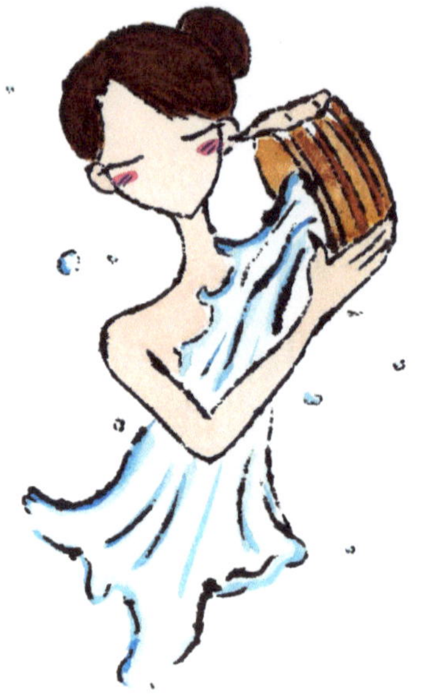

KAKEYU: THE ACTION OF POURING
WARM WATER OVER THE BODY
(MIND YOU, NOT THE HEAD)

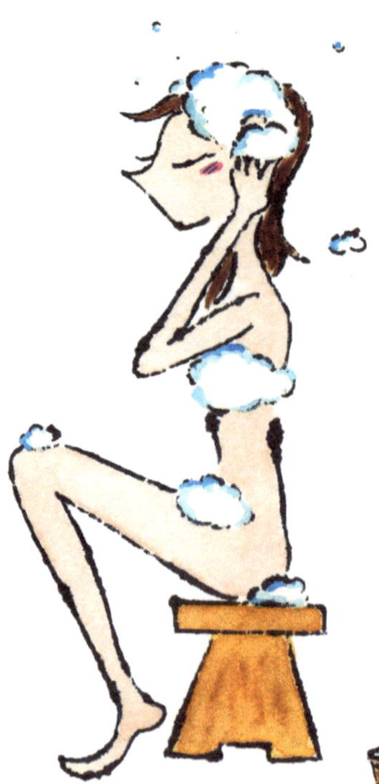

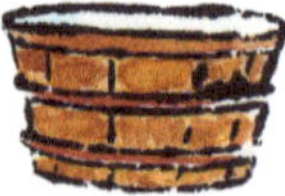

WASHING BEFORE ENTERING
THE ONSEN IS A MUST

you can rinse yourself with the shower head while sitting down on one of the provided wooden stools or if you like, kneeling on the washing area floor. The floors can be of tile, wood, or sometimes stones with drains nearby. Just remember that cleansing yourself while standing is considered bad etiquette, so please refrain from doing so.

You could find a small bath bucket there too, which you can fill with warm water and pour it over your body instead of just using the shower head to rinse yourself. This action of pouring warm water over the body (mind you, not the head) is called *kakeyu* かけ湯, and is a wonderful way to have your body adjusted to the warmer water of an onsen, especially when the temperatures of the changing room, washing area, and the actual baths differs greatly. An unadapted body can get shocked by such temperature differences, which in some cases can result in spasms.

There are people who prefer to quickly wash themselves using the kakeyu method (with makeup removed), go for a short first soak, before washing with soap and shampooing and soaking. However, given the number of face, body and hair products both men and ladies use these days, and after the long trip that is usually required to get to an onsen, fully cleansing yourself first is more refreshing and hygienic.

Now that you have fully cleansed yourself, you are ready to enjoy Japanese hot springs!! There are certain things to keep in mind when soaking in an onsen. You should NOT: emerge your head/hair into the water, use a towel to wrap around your body while soaking, jump into the water, swim, make big splashes, nor speak overly loud. An onsen is a place to relax and refresh oneself, and disturbances are generally not warmly welcomed. For newcomers to onsens, it may seem that there are many rules to follow, but for Japanese people this is common sense and most do so naturally without second thought. I believe that once you have experienced an onsen, you too would come to understand the reasoning behind the manners and customs.

Soaking—Water & Location
About soaking, it is common that there will be at least a couple of onsen baths in a bathing area. The main difference between them is usually the water temperature—one being warmer than the other. Other frequent differences between the baths are: location, i.e. open-air (*rotenboro* 露天風呂) versus indoors (*uchiburo* 内風呂), depth, water mineral content, the material the baths are made of (wood, rocks, tiles and etc.), and if there are any water jet outlets.

Soaking—Temperature & Duration

Onsen is known for its relaxation benefits, not only for the body, but also for the soul. It is a unique experience that cannot truly be replicated elsewhere, and everyone wants to relish this for as much as they can. There is a common misconception even amongst some Japanese, that the water you soak in must be hot and the longer you soak, the better. However, this is not the case. Though hot springs have "hot" in its name, hot springs is not a sauna, and soaking in overly hot, high temperature water and sweating is not the point. The philosophy is that in order to warm up the body from "inside out," soak in lower temperature water of around 37°C to 40°C (98.6°F to 104°F) for a longer period of time (for example 15 minutes) rather than a higher temperature one of 41°C to 42°C (105.8°F to 107.6°F) (for 3 minutes), which is said to "warm up only the surface". Because of the importance of temperature and soaking duration, I will further discuss this in the special section dedicated to this subject: Water temperature & the body, and other benefits of taking a longer lower temperature bath in Chapter 2, page 31.

Depending on the temperature of the water, personal preferences, and body conditions, the soaking time differs greatly. Interesting enough, what Japanese people consider lukewarm or lower temperature water may be high for people of other cultures. The average daily bathwater temperature for Japanese is 40°C to 41°C (105.8°F to 107.6°F), whereas for European and Americans, it is 36°C to 39°C (96.8°F to 102.2°F).[7] Please see Figure 3 on then next page that compares at what temperatures do Japanese and Germans consider bathing water to be lukewarm, comfortable, hot, and extremely hot (and no at all suitable for bathing!). As you can see there is a noticeable difference between the two, and do note that there is a overlap for the Japanese in the "Comfortable" section, as they feel "comfortable" in taking both lukewarm and hot water baths.

That said, start slow and low.

For the purpose of this book, lukewarm or low temperature water will 37°C to 40°C (98.6°F to 104°F) and hot or high temperature is 41°C to 42°C (105.8°F to 107.6°F). Any higher than 42°C (107.6°F) is extremely hot, and is water that bathers will have to enter with much caution.

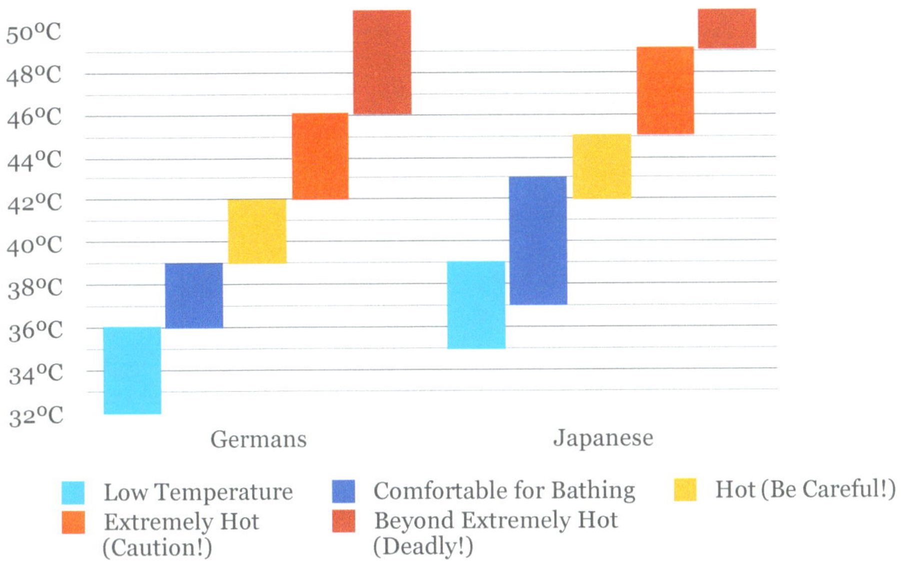
BATHING WATER TEMPERATURE AVERAGES
FOR GERMANS AND JAPANESE IN CELSIUS °C
50°C
48°C
46°C
44°C
42°C
40°C
38°C
36°C
34°C
32°C
Germans
Japanese
Low Temperature
Comfortable for Bathing
Hot (Be Careful!)
Extremely Hot
(Caution!)
Beyond Extremely Hot
(Deadly!)

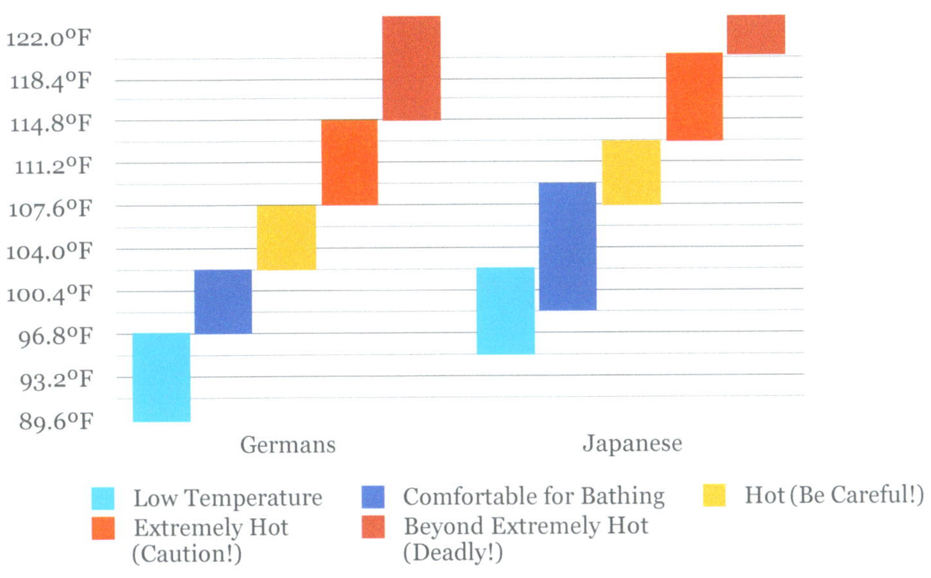
BATHING WATER TEMPERATURE AVERAGES FOR
GERMANS AND JAPANESE IN FAHRENHEIT °F
122.0°F
118.4°F
114.8°F
111.2°F
107.6°F
104.0°F
100.4°F
96.8°F
93.2°F
89.6°F
Germans
Japanese
Low Temperature
Comfortable for Bathing
Hot (Be Careful!)
Extremely Hot
(Caution!)
Beyond Extremely Hot
(Deadly!)

According to advices of medical and onsen associations, including the Ministry of Environment, it is essential that your body slowly adjusts to the temperature and water pressure of an onsen. After washing yourself with soap and shampooing, it is better to:

- First have your body adjusted to the bathing water temperature by pouring water over your body (kakeyu) around 10 times.
- Enjoy the lower temperature baths 37°C to 40°C (98.6°F to 104°F) for 5 to 10 minutes
- Take a short break by slowly getting up from the bath and sitting down somewhere in the bathing area to admire the scenery and atmosphere of the onsen or enjoying kakeyu again
- Re-enter the same or a different low temperature bath for the same amount of time or, if you feel like that your body has already adapted to the temperature, stay a little longer for 15 to 20 minutes
- Please do the above, before moving on to the higher temperature baths 41°C to 42°C (105.8°F to 107.6°F) and only enjoy it for 3 to 10 minutes. For baths over 42°C (107.6°F), please enter with caution and soak for no more than 3 minutes. ***Elderly and persons with high blood pressure, arteriosclerosis, heart disease, or disorders of the respiratory organs should not bathe in water that is 42°C (107.6°F) or higher. Blood thickens under such high temperature and can lead to blood clots***
- Always enter and leave baths slowly[9]

The general rule is the lower the temperature of the water, the longer you can soak in it, but only AFTER your body has adjusted to the onsen temperature. For example, water with a temperature of 37°C to 40°C (98.6°F to 104°F) for 10 to 30 minutes, and 41°C to 42°C (105.8°F to 107.6°F) for 3 to 10 minutes. Of course, this is just a general rule of thumb, and everyone is different. People with medical conditions should always first consult with their doctors to determine what temperatures and duration is best suited for them. Again, I must stress the importance that the elderly and persons with high blood pressure, arteriosclerosis, heart disease, or disorders of the respiratory system should NOT bathe in water that is 42°C (107.6°F) or higher, and children should never soak in an onsen without supervision of an adult. About the type of temperature you choose, it really is up to the bather and their body condition on that day. It is always important to listen to your body. Regardless of the duration, if you feel any faintness, dizziness, or discomfort at anytime, please slowly get up, sit on the side and then leave the bath. Always rehydrate yourself with plenty of warm water or sports drinks after.

Soaking—The Onsen Mark ♨

Besides signifying on maps where onsens and sentos are located, the ♨ mark symbolized the hot water of these places, with the wavy lines representing the steam coming out of the source water, that is embodied by the circle on the bottom. However, there is an other meaning to the ♨ mark that even many Japanese don't know. The three wavy lines are also indicators on how long you should soak in order to get the most out of an onsen bath. It is a difficult to tell from the digitalized mark, but from the original one recognized by the Japanese government in 1948, the left line is slightly shorter than the middle one, and the right one being shortest—this reflects what was the recommended duration for each soak: first you start off soaking for 5 minutes (represented by the left line), then 8 minutes (center line), and last of all, 3 minutes (right line) to wrap up an onsen bath.[10] This again reinforces the fact that long soaks are not the purpose of taking an onsen bath. Instead, it is the slow adaption of the body to the temperature and pressure of the onsen water, and the gradual warming of the body that makes the experience most beneficial.

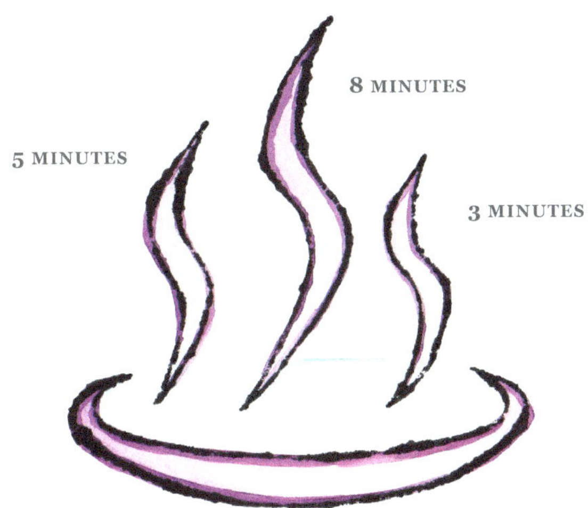

THE ONSEN MARK DOES NOT ONLY REPRESENTS THE LOCATIONS OF HOT SPRINGS, BUT EACH OF ITS WAVY LINE ALSO REPRESENTS HOW LONG A PERSON SHOULD SOAK FOR

Half-Body Soaks

A half-body soak (*hanshinyoku* 半身浴) is one where the water comes up to middle of the soaker's waistline, whereas a full-body soak is where the water comes up to a soaker's collar bone. For the elderly, and people with heart conditions and other disorders related to the respiratory system, it is advised that you enjoy half-body soaks rather than a full-body soak, because half-body soaks are said to put less pressure on your body making it feasible for you to enjoy an onsen too.[11]

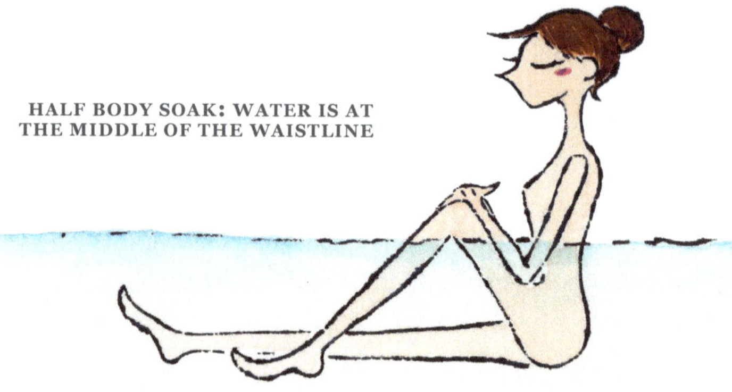

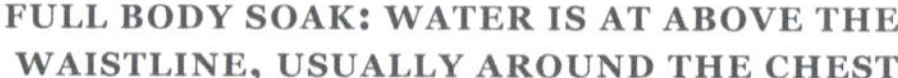

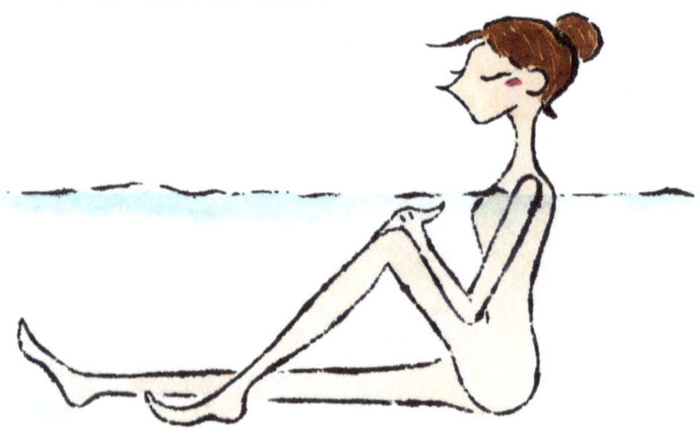

You can do so, but choosing a shallower onsen if one is available, or by sitting on the steps of one, allowing the water only to come up to your waistline. Of course, do this with care, and don't forget to keep your upper body warm, especially during the colder seasons!

On top of the relaxation benefits, if the water contains certain minerals as listed in Figure 1 on page 10, it can help soften the skin, or have other medical properties. A note to keep in mind is that not all minerals will agree with your skin and or body. So if in any case you feel your skin becoming irritated, please do stop soaking in the onsen and rinse off you body with water immediately in the washing area.

After Soaking—Drying, Moisturizing, Hydration, and Relaxation
Now, after soaking in an onsen, it is important not to take a shower again especially if the minerals from the water are good for the skin. Otherwise it would be a waste to rinse off all the wonderful minerals nourishing the skin, unless, as mentioned earlier when the minerals do not agree with your skin, you should rinse off your body with water immediately. Some people would quickly rinse off their feet before heading into the changing room to change. In either case, try to dry yourself off a little with your towel and use the bathroom mat, so that you don't enter the changing room dripping in water.

Noteworthy: it is necessary to completely dry yourself off with the towels provided. If not, the leftover moisture would evaporate, and along with it will be the heat from

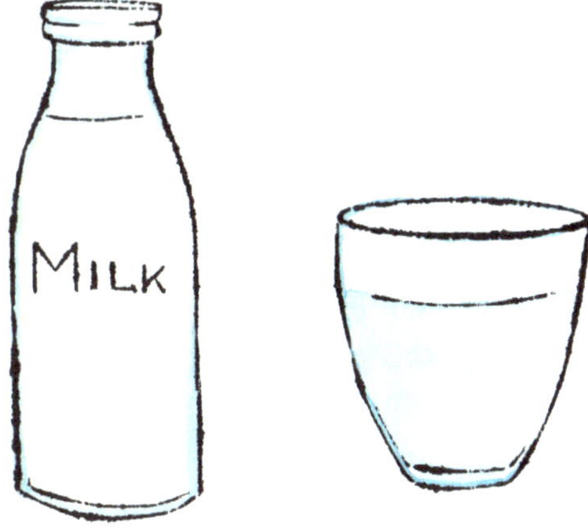

your body. In order to prevent this lost of heat, drying the body thoroughly after leaving an onsen is highly recommended. This can also prevent the possibility of catching colds caused by the rapid warming and cooling of the body, since the temperature of the onsen and the changing room is different, particularly in the winter season. Depending on the ryokans, some have the central heating systems that we are so used to having in North America or Europe, but this is not always the case. Doing so will also keep your core warmer for an extended period of time. This is considered as "lasting warmth" of the core. Though you might not easily feel it because your surface body temperature is not much higher than before soaking in an onsen, this lasting warmth of the core remains after you leave the bath. Hence, soaking for a longer duration in lower temperature water is more common and recommended. Again, lovers of high temperature baths should only soak for a short period of time.

Once you have dried yourself off, be sure to moisturize right away! This is the best time for moisturizing products to be absorbed into your skin, while preventing the wonderful moisture you have gained from soaking in the onsen escaping from your face and body. Try to do so within 5 minutes of leaving the bath because after this time is when the skin starts to lose moisture, and if you don't apply any moisturizing products, your skin will in 20 to 30 minutes become drier than even before you entered the bath![12]

You are now ready to put on your clothes and enjoy the rest of your day! People who are lucky enough to be provided *yukata* 浴衣, the Japanese style bathing robe that looks similar to that of a kimono, can wear it to go outside of the bathing area. Because the provided yukata is usually made of cotton, light in weight, and breathes well, it helps the skin retain just the right amount of moisture and heat after a nice warm bath. A quick and important note on putting on a yukata: the left side must be overlapping the right one. Wearing Japanese robes with the right side overlapping the left, no matter if it is a yukata or kimono, is reserved only for people who have passed away. Now that you have the yukata on the correct way, secure it in place with the *obi* 帯, sash.

After dressing, it is also important to rehydrate yourself with plenty of fluids. There is a common image Japanese frequently associate with after taking a bath—that is, drinking a glass bottle of cold milk or a can of beer. Although you can often find both

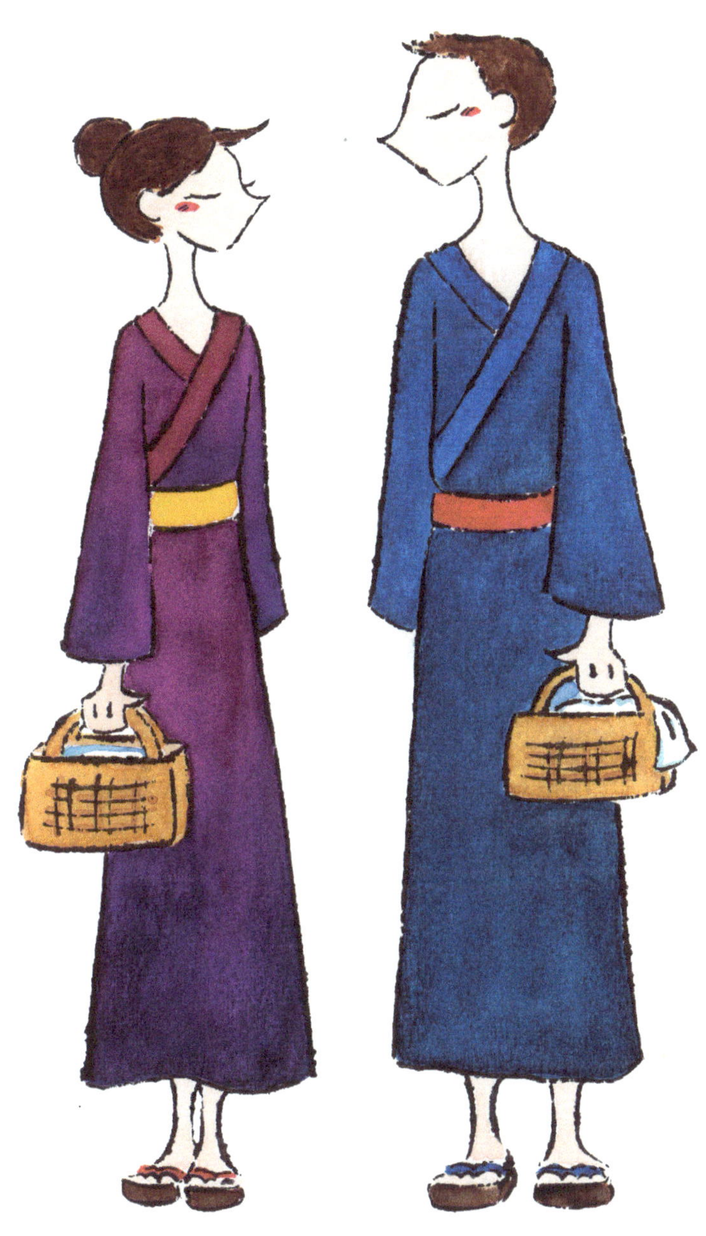

for sale along with other drinks just outside the changing area at the onsen or public bath, *sento* 銭湯, water is probably the best choice. And if you have poor blood circulation or often have cold hands and feet, it is nice to have some warm water or tea instead. This way, you can keep your core temperature high—one of the main reasons for taking a bath in the first place. If you really want to try having a bottle of milk, do so after relaxing for a bit. At some places, you might even find a foot bath, *ashiyu* 足湯, just outside the bathing area, where bathers relax together after a bath. Remember, giving yourself plenty of time to relax after soaking in a bath is big part of onsen experience. A minimum of a 30 minute period is ideal.

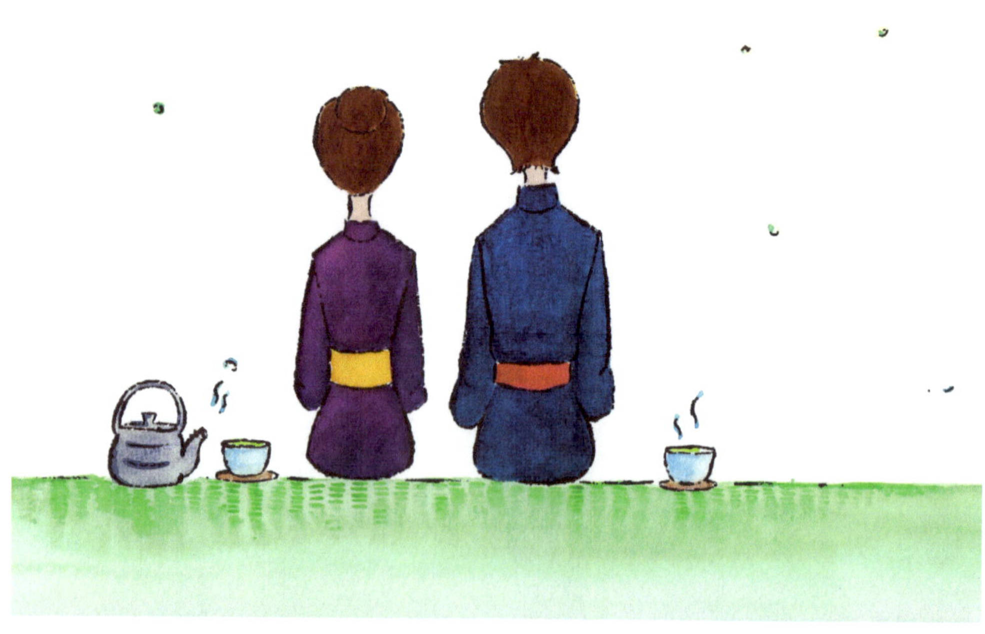

RELAXING AFTER IS A BIG PART OF THE ONSEN EXPERIENCE, A MINIMUM OF 30 MINUTES IS IDEAL

When Not to Enjoy an Onsen

According to The Japan Health & Research Institute, along with and many other medical associations and doctors, you should NOT soak in an onsen:

- After consuming alcohol (alcohol can cause changes in your blood pressure, and bathing after consuming alcohol can result in fainting, dehydration and in some severe cases, strokes)
- Right after or before a meal. Please give yourself 30 to 60 minutes before entering an onsen (bathing has effects on the blood, skin, and kidneys, which can worsen digestion and absorption when soaking with a full stomach)
- Right after or before exercising. Please give yourself 30 to 60 minutes before entering an onsen (bathing right after or before exercising can make it harder for muscles to relax and can place a greater burden on your heart)
- If you are not feeling well, or have a cold and or fever
- Elderly and persons with high blood pressure, arteriosclerosis, heart disease, or disorders of the respiratory system should not bathe in water that is 42°C (107.6°F) or higher
- Children should always be under adult supervision
- People with the following conditions should avoid onsen:
    - Advanced rheumatoid arthritis
    - Colds or other acute illnesses (fever)
    - Cancer, leukaemia, sarcoma
    - Acute communicable disease
    - Serious high blood pressure or arteriosclerosis
    - Serious diabetes
    - Serious heart disease or kidney disease
    - If you have recently experienced cerebral haemorrhage or gastroduodenal ulceration
    - Large vessel aneurysm
    - If you are in the early or late stages of pregnancy

In addition, the following people should avoid sulphur springs:
- The elderly
- People with dry skin, or extremely sensitive skin (especially people with photodermatosis)[13]

ENJOYING SENTOS "PUBLIC BATH"

Public baths or *sento* 銭湯, became popular amongst Japanese during the Edo period (1603 to 1867), and though they have been through many transformations, they remain a big part of the Japanese bathing culture. The number of sentos may have declined after the popularization of having a bathtub in each household, nowadays, you can still have a sento or two in a certain area of town. There are 2,803 registered traditional sento (not the super-sento [large facility sento] or resorts) in Japan as of 2012 and 645 of them are in Tokyo as of 2013.[14]

The etiquette and general guidelines of using a sento is similar to that of an onsen, so please refer to the above pages. The main difference is that yukata and towels are usually not provided, since people would normally take a bath and either return home or continue on with their day.

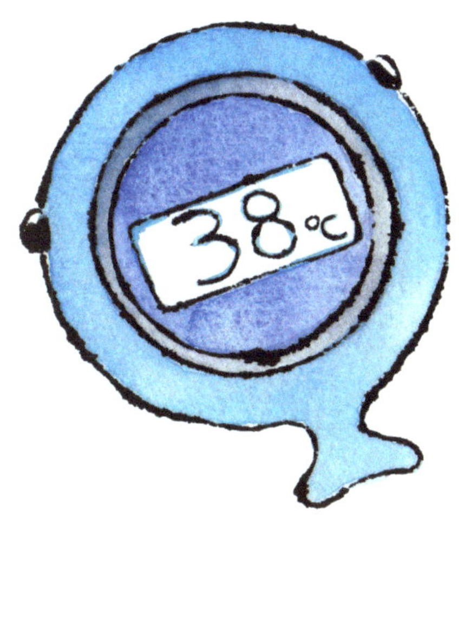

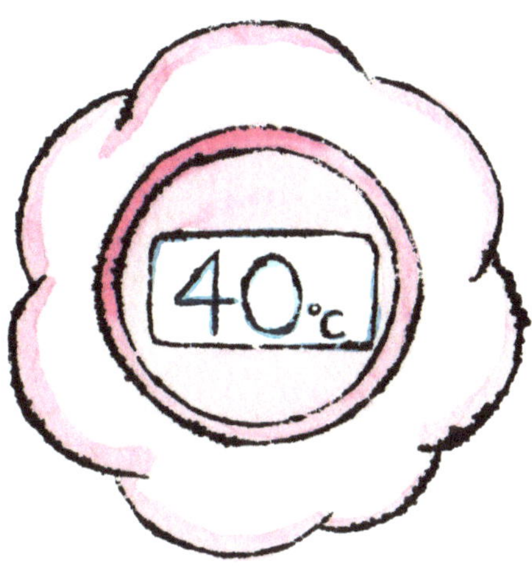

2

WATER TEMPERATURE & THE BODY
AND OTHER BENEFITS OF TAKING A LONGER LOWER TEMPERATURE BATH

We often tend to focus more on the duration of our baths than on what temperature we are soaking in. So, I am dedicating a short and sweet chapter to this factor that is too often overlooked and making it a point of discussion before I introduce how to take a bath wa style at home. Regardless if it is an onsen, sento, or a bath a home, these points apply to all types of bathing.

WARMING AND RELAXATION OF THE BODY—CORE VS OUTER TEMPERATURE

As I noted in the Soaking—Temperature & Duration section of Chapter 1, warming up the body from "inside out" by soaking in lower temperature water of around 37°C to 40°C (98.6°F to 104°F) for a longer period of time (for example 15 minutes) rather than in higher temperature one of 41°C to 42°C (105.8°F to 107.6°F) for less (for 3 minutes), which leads to warming up only "the surface," is key in getting the most out of a wa style bath.

The reason for "inside out" warming is blood usually circulates the body once per minute, and when our blood is warmed up by the bathing water and circulates our body for 15 cycles (based on 1 cycle per minute) the warm blood can reach the smaller blood vessels, which would not have been possible with less cycles, the core of the

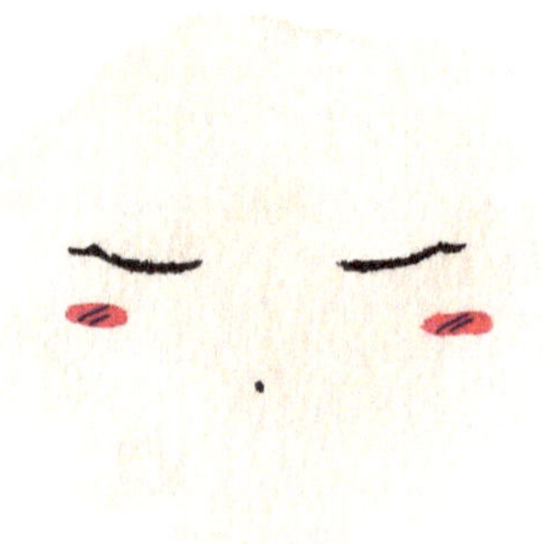

SOAKING IN A TEMPERATURE OF ABOUT 37°C TO 40°C (98.6°F TO 104°F) RELAXES THE BODY

SOAKING IN A HIGH TEMPERATURE OF 41°C TO 42°C (105.8°F TO 107.6°F) CAN HAVE THE OPPOSITE EFFECT

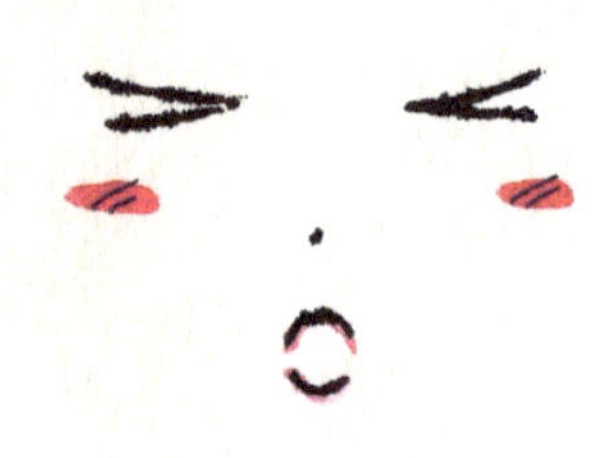

body is too warmed up.[15] Of course, you can warm up the core with high temperature water, but as mentioned before, it is best to avoid soaking in 41°C to 42°C (105.8°F to

107.6°F) water for over 10 minutes. Also, with "surface warming" by high temperature water, heat dissipates from the body quickly, making the cool down process much faster than if a person takes a longer lower temperature bath. So, if you are looking to warm up your body inside out, it is recommended that you soak a little longer in a lower temperature water.

Another reason that lower temperature water is beneficial, is relaxation. When soaking in water with a high temperature of 42°C (107.6°F), the body gets stimulated and switches the autonomic nervous system into an active fight-or-flight mode, where the heart rate quickens, muscles tighten, and the internal organs functions weaken, making it difficult for the bather to relax.[16] Moreover, when the body is in fight-or-flight mode, blood vessels tightens up, limiting blood circulation which is the opposite of a relaxed body condition.[17] Unless you are looking to simulate yourself, a bath temperature of somewhere between the 37°C to 40°C (98.6°F to 104°F) range is the what you should aim for when putting your body into relax mode. Being in a physically relaxed state will help release the stresses of your body, mind, and soul.

TAKING BATHS AT THE RIGHT TEMPERATURE
IS GOOD FOR THE BODY, MIND & SOUL!

SLEEP AND CORE TEMPERATURE

Now that we have covered how water temperature is directly related to relaxation, let's move on to sleep. Though taking long baths in lower temperature water will warm you up from inside out, it can also help lower your core temperature and induce sleep. This is because while soaking in the water, your core temperature will first slowly increase, reach a peak, and slowly decrease again after a certain amount of time, usually after 13 minutes or so.[18] This gradual decrease of the core temperature by taking a bath is similar to that of sleep, where the body dissipates heat and the core temperature is lowered; and hence, enjoying a long lukewarm bath puts the body into sleep mode, making it easy for you to fall asleep quicker, and sleep better.[19] Since it takes around 13 minutes for the core body temperature to start decreasing, it is best to take a bath of at least 20 minutes and an hour or two before bedtime.[20] If you are looking to improve your sleep, then you should definitely give this bathing method a try!

OTHER BENEFITS

Besides relaxation and sleep assistance, there are other benefits of taking a bath. Here are a few:

- The body becomes lighter and feels less pressured, and muscles and joints are more relaxed due to the buoyancy effect from the water. If you were to massage or stretch your body inside the water, the viscosity and resistivity of the bathwater would make it more effective
- The skin can detox itself of dirt, oil, leftover makeup, dust particles and other impurities when the pores opens up and floats away during a bath
- Blood circulation is improved through the warming of the core and by the positive effect water pressure has on the body. This can also help boost your metabolism, and make you feel more refreshed[21]

BATHS VS SHOWERS

It is necessary to keep in mind that the advantages introduced in this section are not effective if you were to take showers instead of baths, even if it was of same temperature and the same length of time. Though showers can warm you up, it:

- Mainly warms up the skin/the surface of the body, and takes roughly twice as long as bath to do so
- Only stimulates the surface of the body
- Lacks the buoyancy and water pressure effects of baths
- Cannot warm up the core nor help the body relax (because only the surface is warmed up)

- Cannot help improve blood circulation[22]

On top on this, it has been said that people who have a habit of taking baths are likely to have a higher core temperature in general of approximately 36.5°C (97.7°F), which allows better blood circulation including that of the white bloods cells, a more balanced autonomic nervous system, and better functioning internal organs, leading to a higher immune system.[23] The making of a healthier you!

Given all these merits of taking a bath, it is no wonder the Japanese people have revelled in the delights of onsen and baths for centuries!

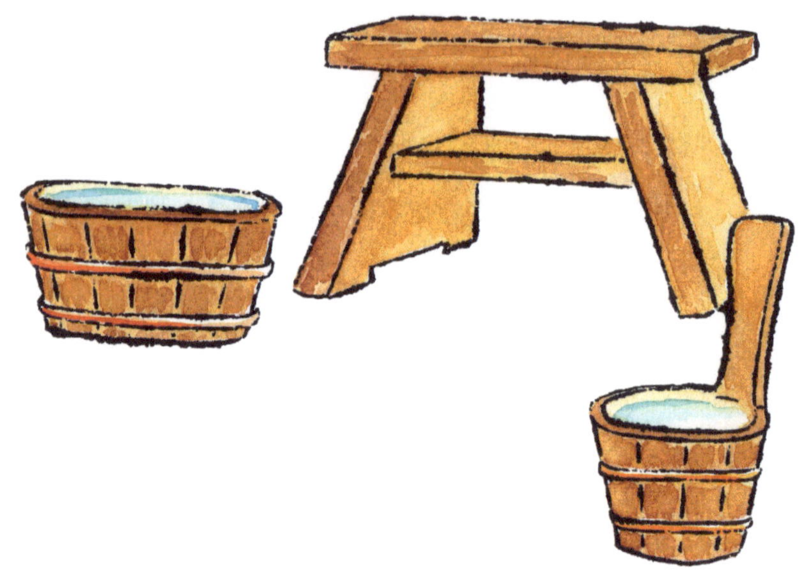

3

THE MODERN JAPANESE BATHROOM & THE IDEAL BATHING ROUTINE

The times have changed, and so has the Japanese bathroom, where in-house bathtubs were not an option for the average person decades ago, now the majority has this little luxury waiting for them to come home to! The bath, bathtub or room, *ofuro*お風呂, holds a very high position in the hearts of many Japanese, and plays an important role in making modern Japanese homes, "home".

THE MODERN JAPANESE BATHROOM

For many Japanese, taking baths is a part of their daily routine, be it at night after a long day or in the morning to refresh themselves prior to checking anything off of their busy schedules. It is important to understand the basic layout or facilities in their bathroom at home can be quite different from that of most Western ones. For example, most Japanese people prefer having the toilet in a separated room from the bathroom, because it is seen as unclean to have to bathe and "do your business" in the same space.

Also, because of their custom of washing before bathing, the shower can be used while the bathtub is full of water. How? The shower head and the bathtub has its own separate faucets, the floor of the entire bathroom is made to handle water with drains, and the doors are waterproof sealed, similar to that of a shower unit, but instead it is bathroom-sized.

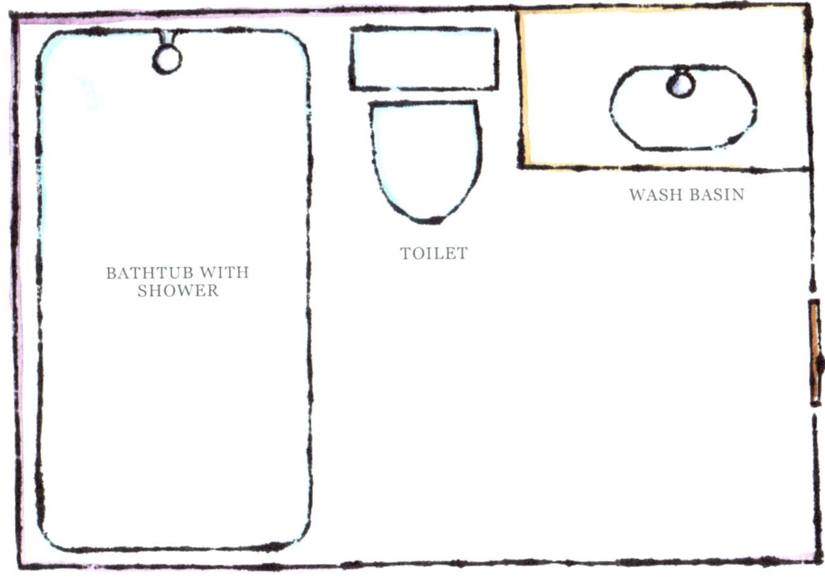

A TYPICAL WESTERN STYLE BATHROOM HAS: A WASH BASIN, TOILET, AND BATHTUB WITH SHOWER ALL IN ONE ROOM

This bathroom is actually a room inside of the real "bathroom," which houses: the bathtub & shower (in a room), a wash basin, and often the laundry machine. And nearby, is where the toilet with a mini wash basin is located.

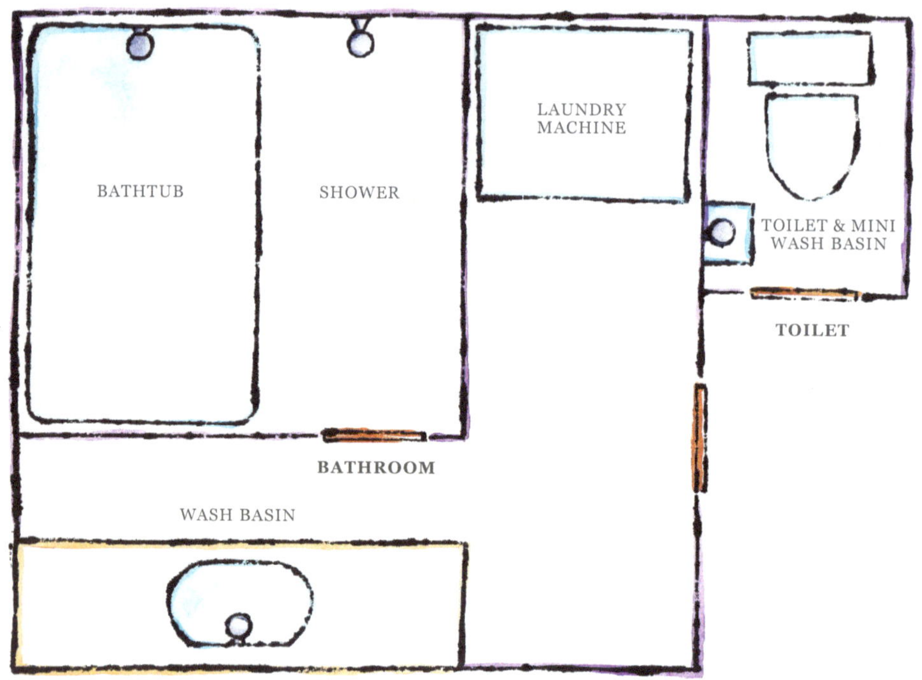

JAPANESE "BATHROOM" WITH A BATHROOM INSIDE

A TYPICAL MODERN JAPANESE STYLE BATHROOM AREA, WHERE THE ACTUAL BATHTUB AND SHOWER ARE IN A ROOM INSIDE OF THE "BATHROOM" WHICH HAS A WASH BASIN, AND OFTEN A LAUNDRY MACHINE. THE TOILET IS IN A SEPARATE ROOM WITH A MINI WASH BASIN

THE IDEAL BATHING ROUTINE

Because of the possibility to shower and then immediately soak in a fully filled bathtub or vice versa, the ideal bathing method recommended by two of Japan's well known university professors and Balneology (which according to the Oxford Dictionary, is the study of medicinal springs and the therapeutic effects of bathing in them) specialists, Dr. Shinya Hayasaka and Dr. Osamu Urushibata, calls for bathers to enter and re-enter the bathtub to soak during their bath time. The following is ideal routine devised from a combination of their suggested steps:

1. Rehydrate by drinking water and start filling your bathtub with water at the desired temperature. Use a bathwater thermostat to help you get the exact desired temperature

2. Remove your makeup and quickly rinse the body using the shower, starting from the feet up

3. Can start soaking in the bath when it is half full, remember to slowly immerse yourself into the water

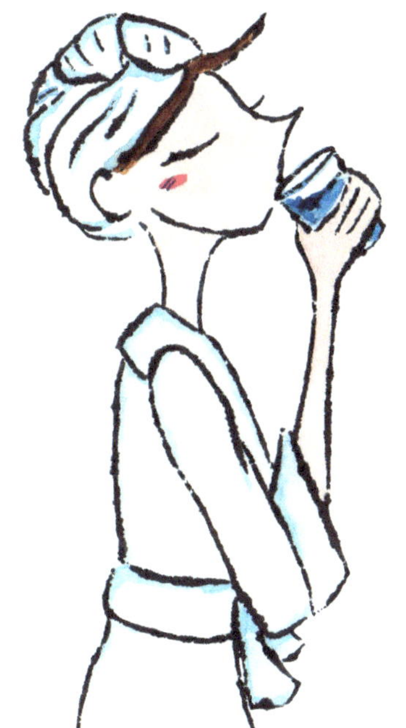

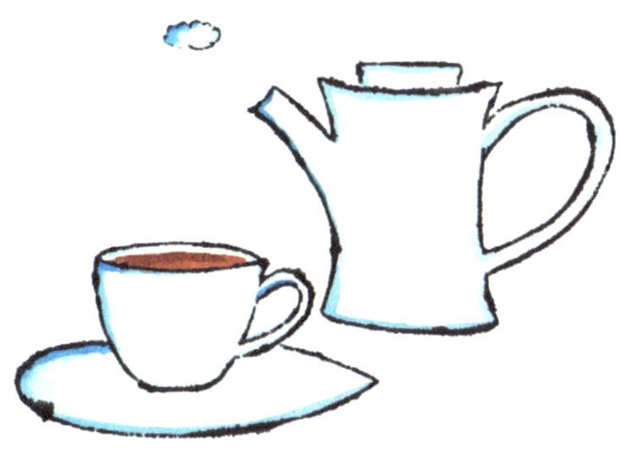

4. While soaking, run the water until it is full, and soak for the desired time (approximately 10 to 20 minutes)

5. Shower again, this time washing your hair and body with gentle mild soap. Avoid using any harsh soaps, scrubs, or towels, and rubbing hard against your skin. Since the human skin is delicate, it should be treated as such with loving, delicate care

6. Ease your body back in, re-enter the bathtub for a short soak (approximately 3 minutes)

7. Slowly get up, dry yourself thoroughly, and apply moisturizer within 5 minutes of leaving the bath

8. Dress warmly

9. Rehydrate by drinking warm water or herbal tea

10. Relax for at least 30 minutes[24]

Am sure you are thinking to yourself right now, "How is this possible to do in my own bathroom?" and might even want to shut close this book. Please don't give up just yet, as I would show you how it is possible in the next chapter: How to take a bath *wa* style at your own home.

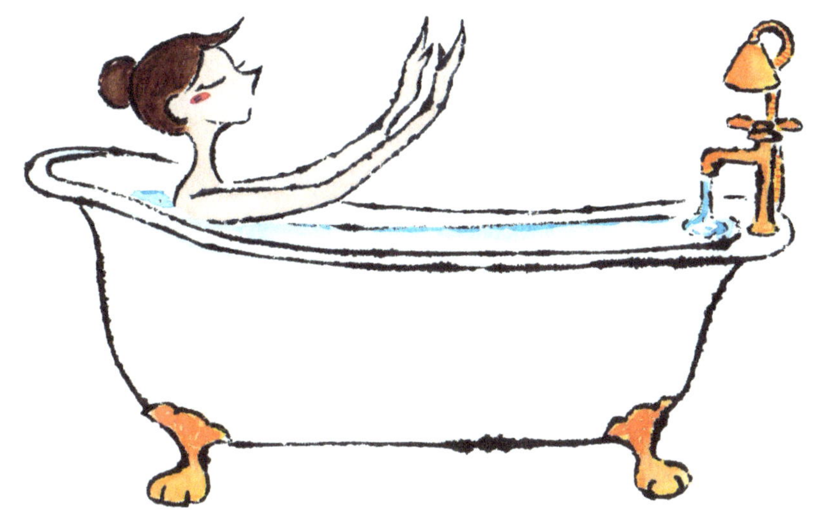

4

HOW TO TAKE A WA STYLE BATH AT THE COMFORTS OF YOUR OWN HOME

What is "wa" style? *Wa* 和 when used in combination form means "Japanese" style, method, or way. When used by itself *wa* 和 can mean peace, friendship and harmony, these elements are essential to a healthy, fulfilling and well-balanced lifestyle. For countless Japanese and now even me, taking a *wa* style bath is not just a habit, it is a part of their being, and for that, their wellbeing. *Wa* style baths can warm us to the core, allow us to relax and release the stress from our everyday lives, make us feel

41

refreshed, while helping our skin detox itself and improve our blood circulation, metabolism, and immune system.

So, how can we take advantage of this centuries-old Japanese wisdom, passed down on to many generations and apply it to our modern, Westernized everyday life, bathroom layout included?   Having grown up in the modern Western society that often takes fast, quick, and efficient over anything else, I came up with some simple, easy to follow steps that may help you with this—well, it is the main purpose of this book. Of course, I did not invent this method, and will not take credit for it. I came up with it after hearing stories and advices from my Japanese friends and doctors (since taking a bath is second nature to them), doing research online, reading books, watching TV, but most of all, after taking lots and lots of baths, i.e. trial-and-error. I want to share with you what I personally have been doing myself on a regular basis, because my bathroom in Tokyo right now is American in layout (meaning the toilet, bathtub, and sink are in the same room; the shower head and bathtub faucet are attached as one unit; the floor has no drains; and the room is not waterproof sealed). I hope you too will enjoy and reap the benefits of taking baths *wa* style at the comforts of your own home.

I am offering two options here: **Evening Option**, and **Morning Option**. See which one suits you the best, and then try to adapt it to your usual routine. It is said that habits takes 3 months to form (even longer for good ones)[25], so don't feel stressed if it seems impossible at first. Take it easy, and enjoy taking a bath when you can. If everyday is not feasible, try once or twice a week, and slowly increase it to whatever works best with your lifestyle and schedule. Of course, if your bathroom is similar to that of a modern Japanese one, please feel free to follow the Ideal Bathing Routine that was introduced in the previous chapter of this book, on page 38. For either option, don't forget to turn on the ventilation fan inside the bathroom.

I. EVENING OPTION

1. After removing all makeup, take a quick and warm shower of around 37°C to 41°C (98.6°F to 105.8°F) depending on your personal preference. I am adding an extra 1°C, because the air around the shower tends to cool down the water a bit easier than that of a bath. Use soap, and shampoo (if needed). Long showers of over 15 minutes are not recommended, as you will be taking a bath soon after

2. Dry yourself thoroughly and wrap yourself in a fluffy robe or towel after taking the shower

3. Apply toner or a light lotion on your face. It's a great time for the product to be absorbed by the skin, and it also prevents the skin for dehydration. Note, leave the full moisturizing routine (facial serums, creams and body products until after taking the bath)

4. Quickly rinse off the leftover residue/soap bubbles from the bathtub, and fill the tub with water ideally between 37°C to 40°C (98.6°F to 104°F) depending on the season, your personal preference, and body condition. I suggest trying, but it's not a rule:
37°C to 39°C (98.6°F to 102.2°F) for Summer
38°C to 40°C (100.4°F to 104°F) for Winter

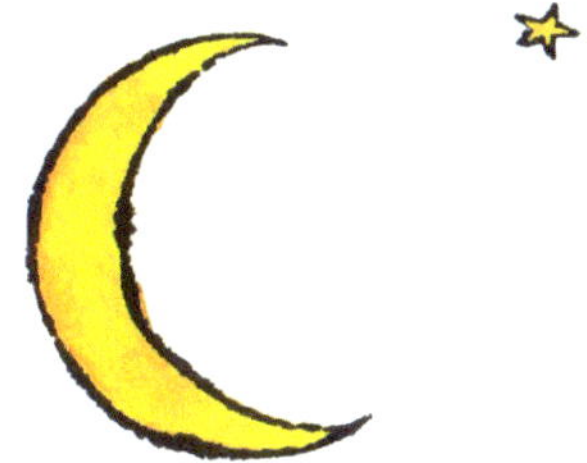

Because the temperature water is hard to tell just by testing with your hands, it is recommended that you get a bathwater thermometer. There are many out there on the market, especially for babies. Even though in many parts of Asia, there is a water boiler for the bathroom with the thermostat showing the temperature of the water being ran, I still find having a floating thermometer inside the tub, to be much more accurate, since the water temperature can be affected by the temperate of the air when coming out of the faucet. I have a handy digital thermostat that comes with a timer.

5. While waiting for the tub to fill, go out of the bathroom and have a glass of water warm or at room temperature. You might also want to bring some water into the bathroom, just in case you feel a little dehydrated while soaking in the bath. Of course, to avoid dangerous broken glass situation, pour the water in a shatter-free cup or bottle please

6. Once the bathtub is filled to 40%, you can take off your towel or robe and slowly immerse your body into the water and start to enjoy soaking. Continue to allow the water to run, until it is 80% to 85% full (over 90% is not suggested, since it increases the chances of a overflowing tub, and that cause a lot of trouble)

7. Recommended soaking time for 37°C to 40°C (98.6°F to 104°F): 10 to 20 minutes. For people who are just starting to take a bath, you should begin with a lower temperature (37°C to 38°C or 98.6°F to 100.4°F) and shorter duration (5 to 10 minutes), and slowly increase it to your own liking after your body has gotten used to baths. If you find it difficult to just relax and do nothing in the bathtub during this time, you can:

   - Listen to music (from a audio source that is either waterproof, or coming from outside of the bathroom—please don't use your mobile phone or MP3 players while taking a bath! It's too dangerous in many senses)
   - Give your body a nice massage inside the water or even stretch out your body, since the viscosity and resistivity of the bathwater make it more effective

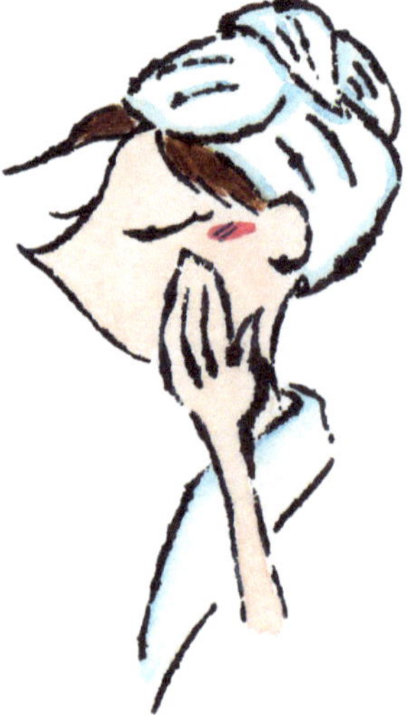

MOISTURIZING WITHIN 5 MINUTES OF
GETTING OUT OF THE BATH IS ESSENTIAL

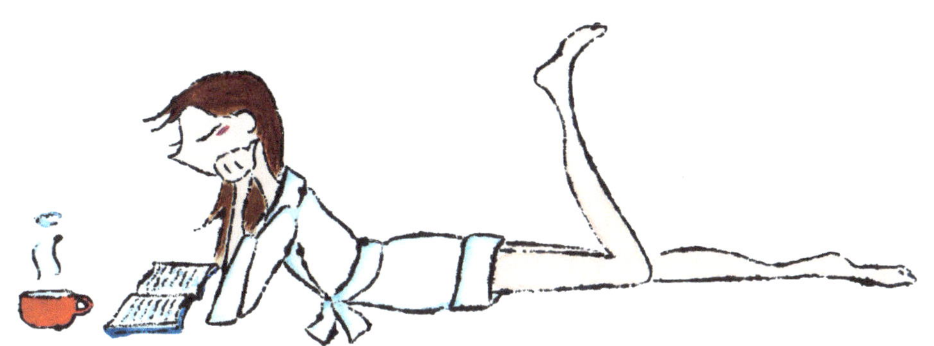

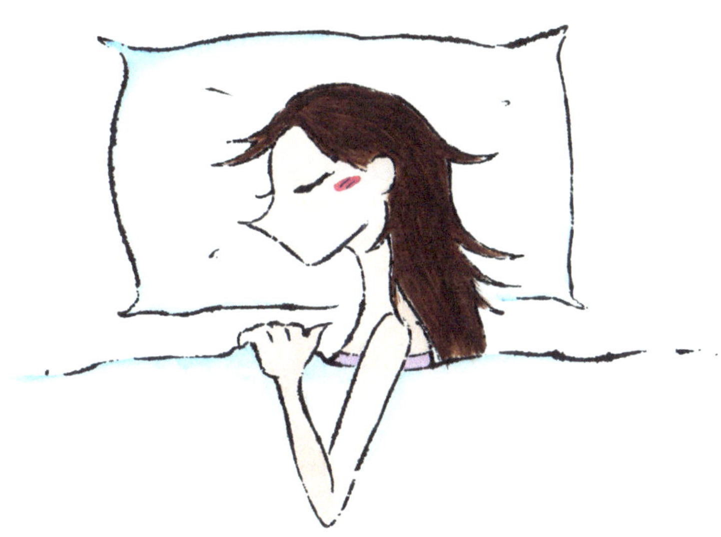

RELAXING FOR A BIT AND SLEEPING WITHIN **1.5** HOUR AFTER A BATH IS BEST

8. When you are done soaking, slowly get up from the bathtub and dry yourself thoroughly. Once again, apply toner or light lotion on your face immediately, but this time follow with other moisturizing facial products (serums, creams) and then products for the body. Try to moisturize within 5 minutes of getting out from the bath

9. Dress warmly enough to maintain you newly gained warmth from the bath

10. Drink some water or other fluids, such as herbal tea to keep yourself hydrated. Avoid fluids that are cold, because you want your body temperature, including the core to be stable

11. Now is a good time to blow dry your hair, if needed

12. Relax for 30 minutes or so. If possible, sleep soon afterwards, with an hour or an hour and a half. Sweet dreams!

II. MORNING OPTION

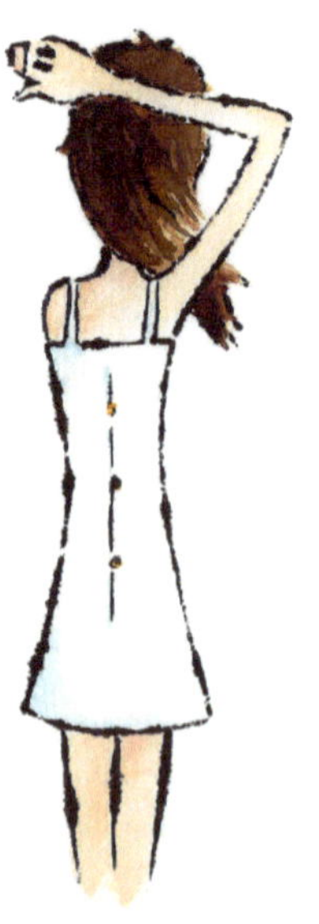

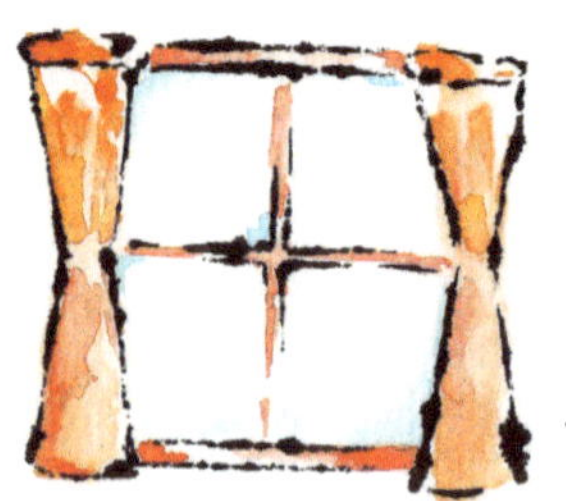

MORNING BATHS IS A GREAT WAY TO START YOUR DAY

As much as I like the Evening Option, I do take more baths in the morning because I am an earlier raiser and I work from home. I feel it is also a more relaxing way to start my day. This maybe not feasible for the many time-strapped people in the morning on a weekday, but it's a great option on a weekend. Please try it sometime and you will know what I mean!

1. Shower at night as usual

2. After waking up and relaxing a bit, you can either take a bath first or have breakfast first and then a bath. However, it is recommended that you wait at least 30 minutes in between doing each. Meaning you can take a bath 30 minutes after having breakfast, or have breakfast 30 minutes after taking a bath. If you tend to have bigger breakfasts, please wait at least 60 minutes in between. The same goes for exercising. Do give yourself a 30 to 60 minutes interval between the two activities. For me, I first have breakfast, read the news or reply some emails which normally takes more than an hour, and then take a bath.

3. Follow the Steps 4 to 12 under the Evening Option

4. You are now ready to enjoy your the rest of your day!

If you have already gotten used to taking high temperature baths for sometime, and are looking for a way to refresh yourself (meaning to stimulate your body) in the morning—say before work, you can try soaking in a 41°C (105.8°F) or 42°C (107.6°F) bathwater, but for NO more than 5 minutes. Do make sure that you have already adapted to such a high temperature bath beforehand and are comfortable with it, as this is higher than the normally recommended one. And don't forget that you still need to give yourself plenty of time to take it easy after your bath.

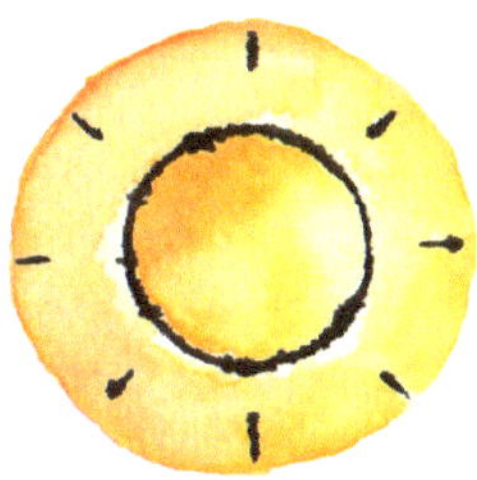

Reminder, regardless of your choice of following the Ideal Bathing Routine, Evening Option, or Morning Option, you should NOT take a bath:

- After consuming alcohol
- Right after or before a meal. Please give yourself a 30 to 60 minutes interval between the activities
- Right after or before exercising. Please give yourself 30 to 60 minutes interval between the activities
- When you feel your body condition is not well

EXTRAS GOODS

There are several things that have been indispensable for me when taking baths, and I think they too would help you make taking wa style bath more enjoyable and easier:

- A bathwater thermometer. There are many on the market for babies, and are perfect for accurately measuring the temperature of your bathwater. There are ones with timers too, and they take the guess work out of the entire process.

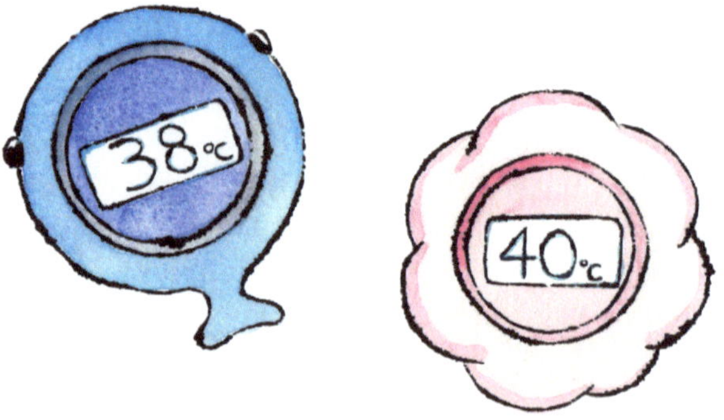

BATHWATER THERMOMETERS ARE VERY HANDY TO HAVE

- Bath salts and other similar bath products. There are many products available, especially here in Japan, which makes taking a bath more relaxing, fun, and enjoyable. It really depends on your personal preference, what product works best for you. In my case, having sensitive skin and nose, I went through many bath products before finding some that worked for me—where some contained too many chemical preservatives and were too strong in scent, while others had too much colouring agent that stains a non-porcelain bathtub or some with essential oils made cleaning the bathtub afterwards a real chore (yes, I am lazy). Of course just like with skincare, once I found the ones I liked, I love taking a bath with them every day! However, I found bubble baths or other products that require showering afterwards were not suitable at all for *wa* style baths and cannot recommend them

- Lightweight cotton or natural fibre bath towels that are absorbent and quick drying. They absorb water from the body quickly, making it easier to thoroughly dry

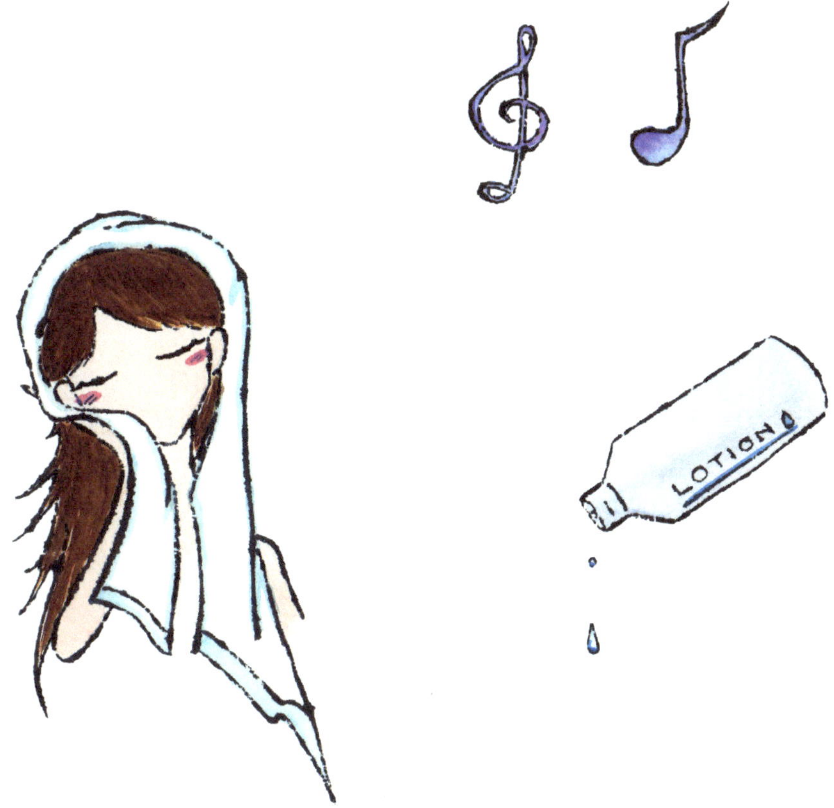

OTHER GREAT THINGS TO HAVE: LIGHTWEIGHT COTTON TOWELS & ROBES, LESS EXPENSIVE & LIGHT LOTIONS OR TONERS, AND OF COURSE, RELAXING MUSIC

yourself and prevent you from catching a cold. And because they are light in weight, the towels themselves dry fast too. I found natural fibers to be softer, generate less static, and last longer even after many years of use, which is perfect for delicate skin.

- A lightweight cotton or natural fibre bathrobe. It comes in handy when you are waiting for the bathtub to be filled after your shower, and when you want to dry and stay warm while moisturizing your face and body quickly after a bath. Being surrounded by a warm, soft, and fluffy bathrobe after a nice long bath is the best feeling! I say lightweight again because heavier bathrobes can make the body feel heavy, which for me defeats the purpose of taking a relaxing bath

- A less expensive light lotion or toner to be applied on your face after taking shower and in between waiting for the bathtub to be filled and your bath. I find that my face tends to get dry during this time, but I don't feel like using an expensive toner before my bath—what a waste! This was the workaround that I found worked for me

- Music. I have a bath time playlist on my laptop, and have it playing (my laptop is never inside the bathroom, but near by in my room) when I am taking bath. it makes the whole experience even more relaxing and delightful. It also works as a timer, say when a certain song begins to play, it's time to slowly get out of the tub

I hope with these two options, their simple steps, and some handy items that you too will come to fall in love with taking *wa* style baths, and see what you thought was once an inconvenience and maybe even a waste of time as a precious, self-caring, part of your wholesome wellbeing instead. It is an experience that you have to experience for yourself. And I say this with all my sincerity, because I too had doubts for the longest time, but have since taken my words back after gaining so much from my *wa* style bathing lifestyle. The aim of me writing this book is to spread the word on this wonderful custom that despite it having a very long history, can be adapted into our modern life and help us make the most out of our every day, which is the true essence of a *wa* style bath!

NOTES

1 Dietitians of Canada, "Your Health, Nutrition A-Z, Water," http://www.dietitians.ca/Your-Health/Nutrition-A-Z/Water.aspx (accessed June 24, 2015).

2 Ministry of Environment, the Government of Japan, "温泉の定義 [Onsen no Teigi/The Definition of Hot Spring]" http://www.env.go.jp/nature/onsen/point/ (accessed June 25, 2015).

3 The Japan Health & Research Institute, "What Types of Onsen Have You Tried?," http://www.jph-ri.or.jp/kenko_f/onsen_english/contents/donoonsen.html (accessed June 25, 2015).

4 HITOU - The Japan Association of Secluded Hot Spring Inns, "What are Onen?," http://www.hitou.or.jp/en/spateaching/spateaching01.html (accessed April 12, 2015).

5 Yasuhiro Ishikawa, お風呂の達人 バスクリン社員が教える究極の入浴術 [*Ofuro no Tatsujin Bathclin Shain ga Oshieru Kyukyoku no Nyuyoku-jutsu/The Ultimate Method of Bathing from the Bathing Expert Employees of Bathclin*] (Tokyo: Soshisha, 2011), 80.

6 Hiroko Ishii, 温泉ビューティー [*Onsen Byuti/Onsen Beauty*] (Tokyo: GreenCat, 2007), 89.

7 Osamu Urushibata, 美しくなる入浴術 [*Utsukushiku Naru Nyuyoku-jutsu/Bathing Methods for Becoming More Beautiful*] (Tokyo: Medical Tribune, 2013), 42 - 43.

8 Yuko Agishi, 温泉と健康 [*Onsen to Kenko/Hot Springs and Health*] (Tokyo: Iwanami Shoten, 2009), 34.

9 Ministry of Environment, the Government of Japan, "あんしん・あんぜんな温泉利用のいろは [Anshin Anzen na Onsen Riyo no Iroha/How to Use Hot Springs Safely and with Peace of Mind]," http://www.env.go.jp/nature/onsen/docs/zentaiban.pdf (accessed June 25, 2015).
The Japan Health & Research Institute, "Things to Keep in Mind," http://www.jph-ri.or.jp/kenko_f/onsen_english/contents/tyui.html, (accessed May 20, 2015).
HITOU - The Japan Association of Secluded Hot Spring Inns, "Recommended Ways to Use Onsen," http://www.hitou.or.jp/en/spateaching/spateaching04.html (accessed June 25, 2015).

10 Hiroko Ishii, 95 - 96.

11 Shinya Hayasaka, たった**1°C**が体を変えるほんとうに健康になる入浴法 [*Tatta 1°C ga Karada o Kaeru Honto ni Kenko ni Naru Nyuyoku-ho/Only 1°C Can Change The Body - The Real Healthy Bathing Method*] (Tokyo: KADOKAWA, 2014), 21.

12 Osamu Urushibata, 50.

13 The Japan Health & Research Institute, "Things to Keep in Mind".

14 NTT TownPage Data, "日本一、お風呂好きの都道府県はどこ？～温泉・銭湯から入浴文化をたどる[Nihon Ichi, Ofuro-suki no Todofuken wa Doko? ~ Onsen Sento kara Nyuyoku Bunka o Tadoru/Which Prefecture Likes Bathing the Most? Tracing the Bathing Culture from Hot Springs to Public Baths]" http://tpdb.jp/townpage/order?nid=TP01&gid&scrid=TPDB_GP01 (accessed June 24, 2015).
Tokyo Sento Association, "東京都内の銭湯の数の推移 [Tokyoto-nai no Sento no Kazu no Suii/Changes in the Number of Public Baths in Tokyo]" http://www.1010.or.jp/menu/sentousu.html (accessed June 24, 2015).

15 Yasuhiro Ishikawa, 78.

16 Shinya Hayasaka, 10 - 11.

17 Yasuhiro Ishikawa, "入浴でカラダ作りお風呂でリカバリー！[Nyuyoku de Karada Tsukuri Ofuro de Rikabari!/Recovering the Body by Bathing!]" Bathclin, https://www.bathclin.co.jp/happybath/sportsvol06q1/ (accessed April 23, 2015).

18 Hiroya Shimasaki, "Analysis of the Thermal Effects of Bathing: Comparison of a Hot Spring Plunge Bath and Home Bathtub Bath," *Japan Health & Research Institute: Annual Research Report* 35 (2014): 32.

19 Yasuhiro Ishikawa, 46 - 47.

20 Shinya Hayasaka, 46.

21 Shinya Hayasaka, 12 - 14.
   Osamu Urushibata, 26.

22 Osamu Urushibata, 24.

23 Toru Abo, "体温免疫力があれば、どんな病気も恐くない！[Taion Meneki-ryoku ga Areba, Donna Byoki mo Kowakunai!/If You Have a Strong Immunity from Body Temperature, You Are Not Afraid of Any Illnesses]", 冷え取り健康ジャーナル **51**号: 入浴美読本 [*Hie Tori Kenko Janaru 51 Go: Nyuyokubi Dokuhon/Getting Rid of Cold Sensitivity Health Journal Issue No. 51: The Bathing Beauty Guidebook*] (Tokyo: Kenko Journal, 2012), 50 - 51.

24 Shinya Hayasaka, 15.
   Osamu Urushibata, 46 - 47.

25 David DiSalvo, *What Makes Your Brain Happy and Why You Should Do the Opposite* (Amherst, NY: Prometheus Books, 2011), 219.

AFTERWORD

Taking baths became a part of my life that I never thought would be this significant. Ask me a few years ago if I would spend this much time on reading, looking for information, and asking people, soaking—enjoyably so, let alone writing a book on baths, I would have said that you were crazy. Fast forward to now, I have dedicated over a year and a half for this project.

When writing this book, I had to narrow down to what I felt was the most relevant to novices and people looking to maximize the benefits of enjoying *wa* style baths. Because the subject of Japanese bathing culture and its virtues is very wide and deep, I have barely skimmed the surface of it. If you found this book interesting, then I encourage you to learn more about it. Since most of the sources of the information presented here was only available in Japanese and a good portion of it is considered common knowledge here in Japan, I have taken extra care in citing them, sources that I found very useful myself (some are available in English).

I am not saying that taking baths is the ultimate cure-all to all and its effectiveness varies among people, but it has definitely made a difference in my own life and I hope more people outside of Japan would come to know of the joys of *wa* style baths. However, more than reading, you should go experience the wonders of *wa* style baths for yourself, and if visiting Japan is impossible, then at least try it at home!

GLOSSARY OF JAPANESE TERMS
IN ORDER OF APPEARANCE

1. 和 *wa*: "Japanese" style, method, or way when used in combination form it means. When used by itself, *wa* 和 can mean peace, friendship and harmony

2. 温泉 *onsen*: Hot spring

3. 浴衣 *yukata*: Japanese bathing robes, often made of light weight natural fibers, such as cotton

4. 銭湯 *sento*: Public baths

5. ♨: Onsen Mark which signifies on maps where onsens and sentos are located

6. 湯 *yu* (sometimes with お in front of it, or sometimes written as ゆ): Hot water

7. 露天風呂 *rotenburo*: Outdoor onsen bath

8. 内風呂 *uchiburo*: Indoor onsen bath

9. 旅館 *ryokan*: Traditional Japanese inn

10. 温泉法 *onsenho*: "Hot Spring Law" created by Japanese government in 1948. Under this law, in order to be officially considered as an onsen, the water from the natural spring must be over 25°C (77°F) degrees in temperature, and have certain amount of natural chemical/mineral content

11. 単純温泉 *tanjun onsen*: Simple spring

12. 二酸化炭素泉 *nisankatansosen*: Simple carbon dioxide spring

13. 炭酸水素塩泉 *tansansuiso ensen*: Bicarbonated earth spring (carbonated)

14. 塩化物泉 *enkabutsusen*: Sodium bicarbonated spring (carbonated)

15. 含よう素泉 *gan yososen*: Chloride spring

16. 硫酸塩泉 *ryusan ensen*: Sulphate spring

17. 含鉄泉 *gan tetsusen*: Ferruginous spring

18. 硫黄泉 *iosen*: Sulphur spring

19. 酸性泉 *sanseisen*: Acidic spring

20. 放射能泉 *hosha nosen*: Radioactive spring

21. 貸切温泉 *kashikiri onsen*: Onsen that bathers to "borrow" for a limited amount of time, so that it can be enjoyed privately

22. 源泉かけ流し *gensen kakenagashi*: Continuous flow from source

23. かけ流し *kakenagashi*: Continuous flow

24. 給湯口源泉・浴槽加温循環 *kyutoguchi gensen - yokuso kaon junkan*: Direct flow from source - heated and circulation bath system

25. 給湯口源泉・浴槽加温・濾過・殺菌循環 *kyutoguchi gensen - yokuso kaon - roka - sakkin junkan*: Direct flow from source - heated, filtered, sterilized, and circulation system

26. 給湯口を含む加温・濾過・殺菌循環 *kyutoguchi wo fukumu kaon - roka - sakkin junkan*: Hot spring supply is heated, filtered and sterilized before entering the bath

27. 大浴場 *dai yokujo*: Bathing area, which consists of: a changing room, washing area, and big baths (open-air bath, indoor bath, or both)

28. のれん *noren*: Japanese short split curtains or curtain dividers

29. 女 *onna:* Woman, female

30. 男 *otoko*: Man, male

31. 混浴 *konyoku*: Unisex bath

32. 脱衣所 *datsui jo:* Changing room

33. 洗い場 *arai ba*: Open communal washing/showering space

34. かけ湯 *kakeyu*: Action of pouring warm water over the body (mind you, not the head). A method of washing and getting the body to adjust to bath water temperatures

35. 半身浴 *hanshinyoku*: Half-body soak is one where the water comes up to middle of the soaker's waistline, whereas a full-body soak is where the water comes up to a soaker's collar bone

36. お風呂 *ofuro:* Bath, bathtub or room

ABOUT THE AUTHOR

Jodi Sam is an illustrator - writer - fashion stylist - daydreamer. Her love for the arts began as a young child. At age twelve, she was featured in Emily Carr's British Columbia Young Artist Exhibition, which toured cities across Western North America. Her work is now a part of the permanent collection of Chicago Children's Museum.

In September 2013 her illustrated book, *My Little Book of Happiness*, was released internationally. After 6 1/2 years in Tokyo, she relocated back to her hometown of Vancouver, Canada in late 2016 and is actively working on her new projects. She decided to write *How to Take a Wa Style Bath* after benefiting greatly from taking Japanese style baths, which has brought relief to her chronic body pain.